Contents

Trace the lines

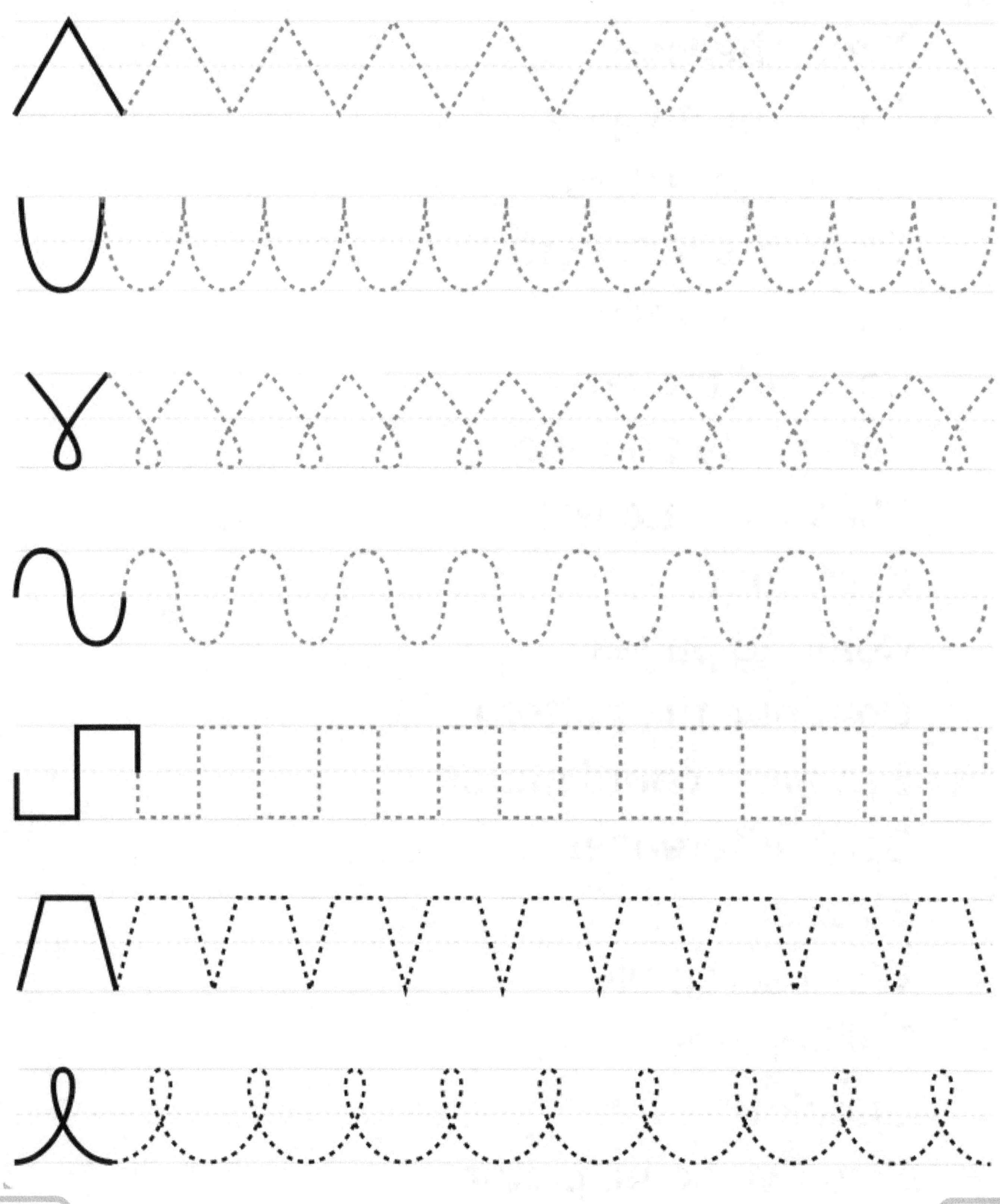

Trace the lines

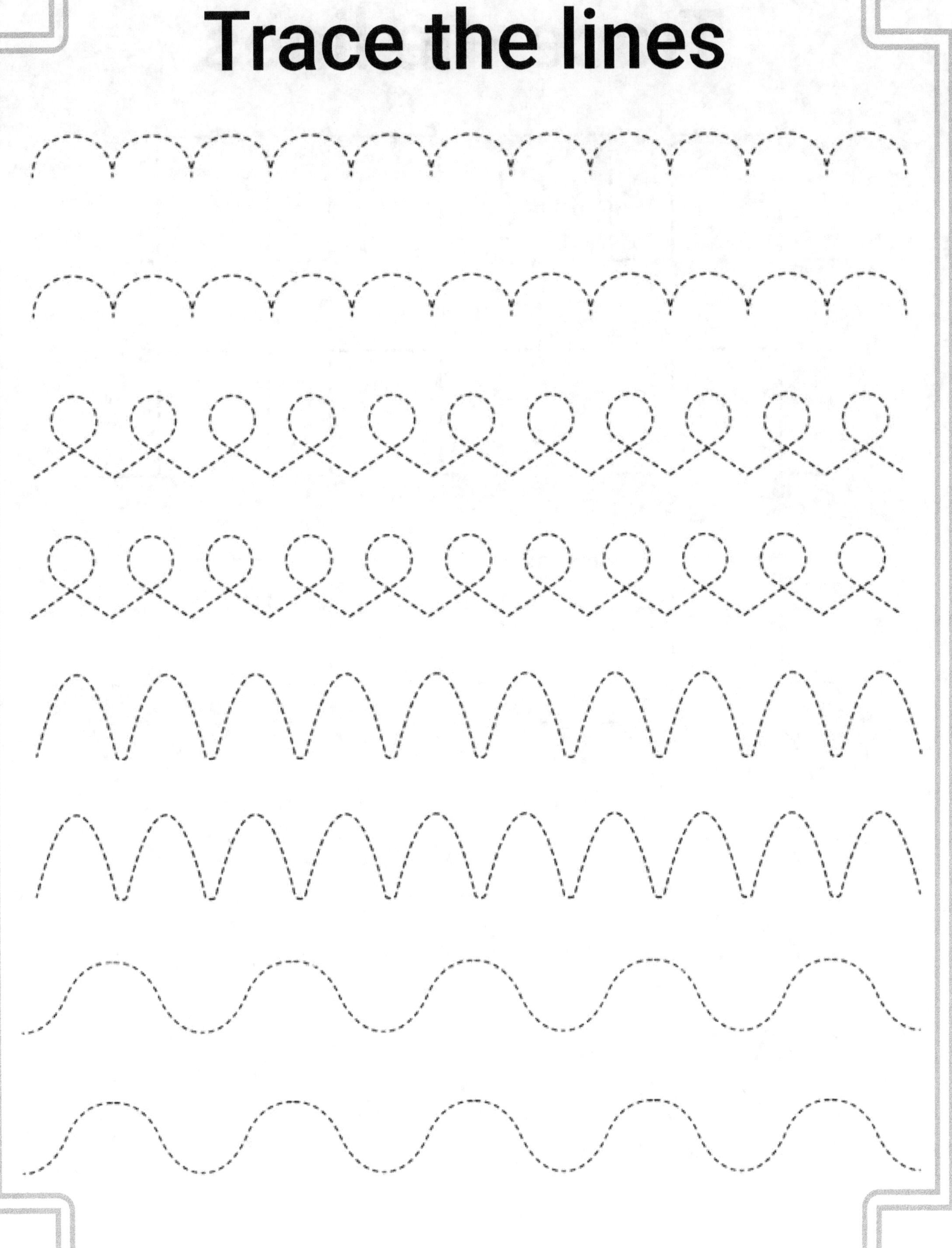

Trace the lines

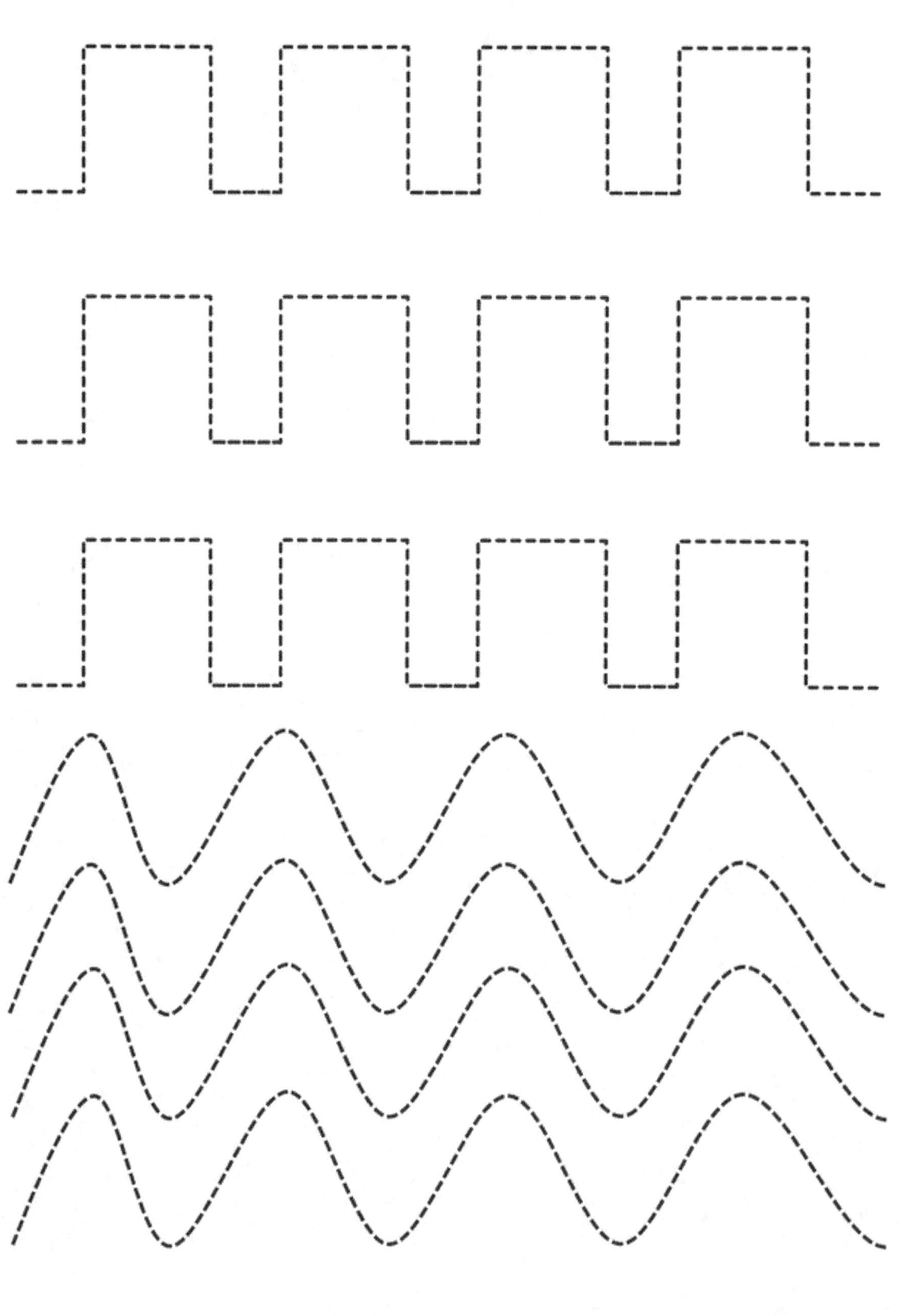

Trace the shapes

Trace the shapes

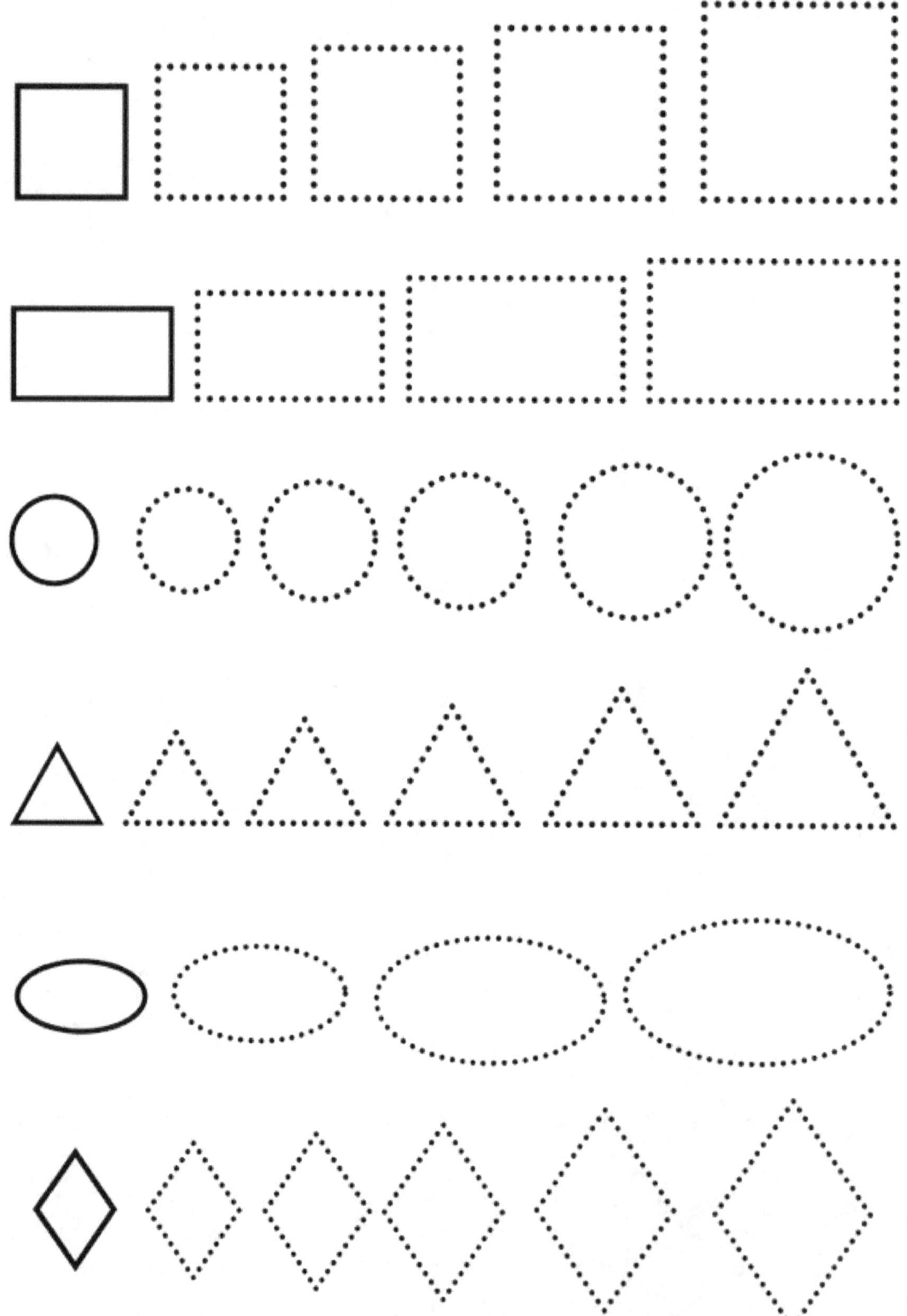

Trace the shapes

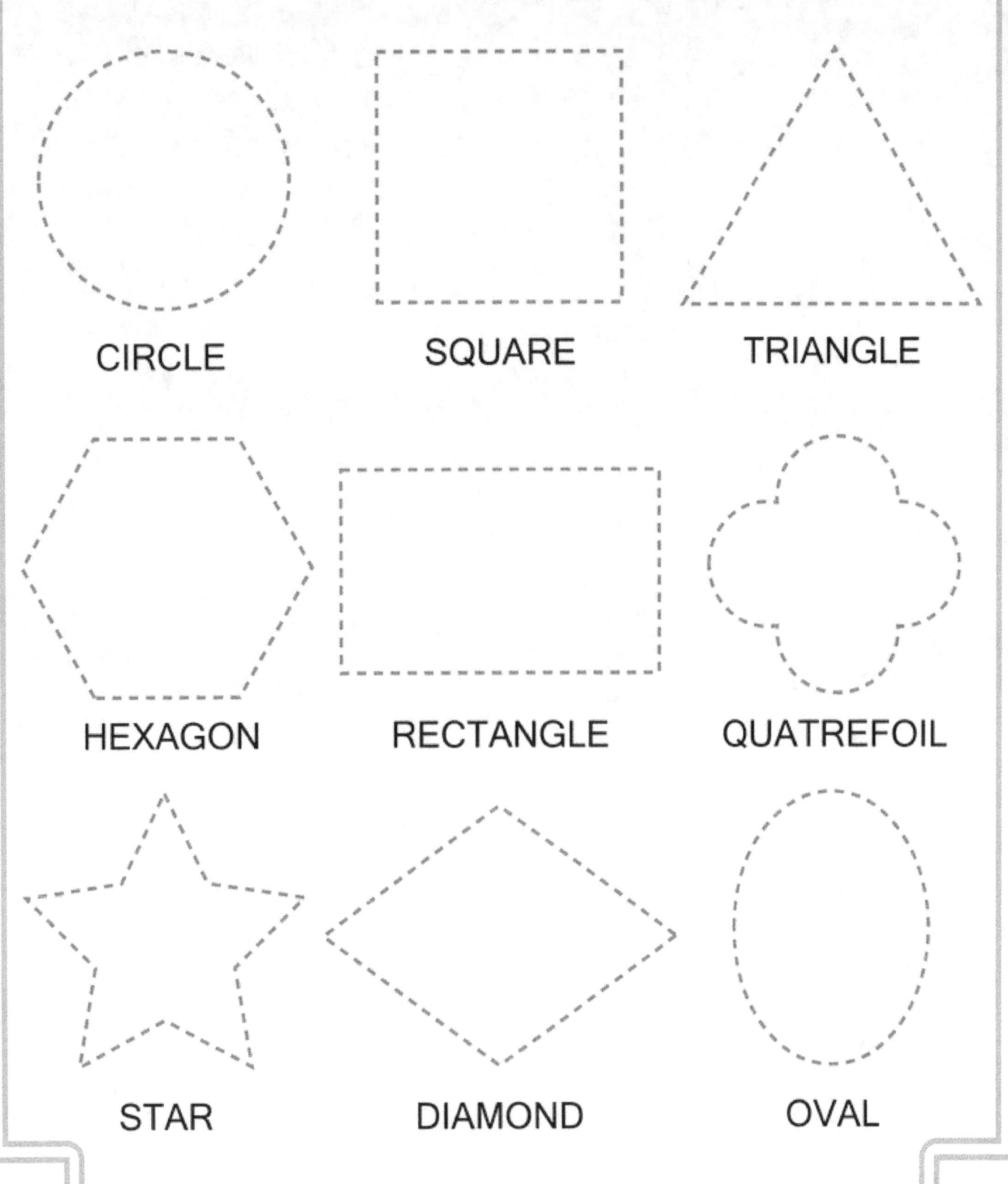

Trace the letters

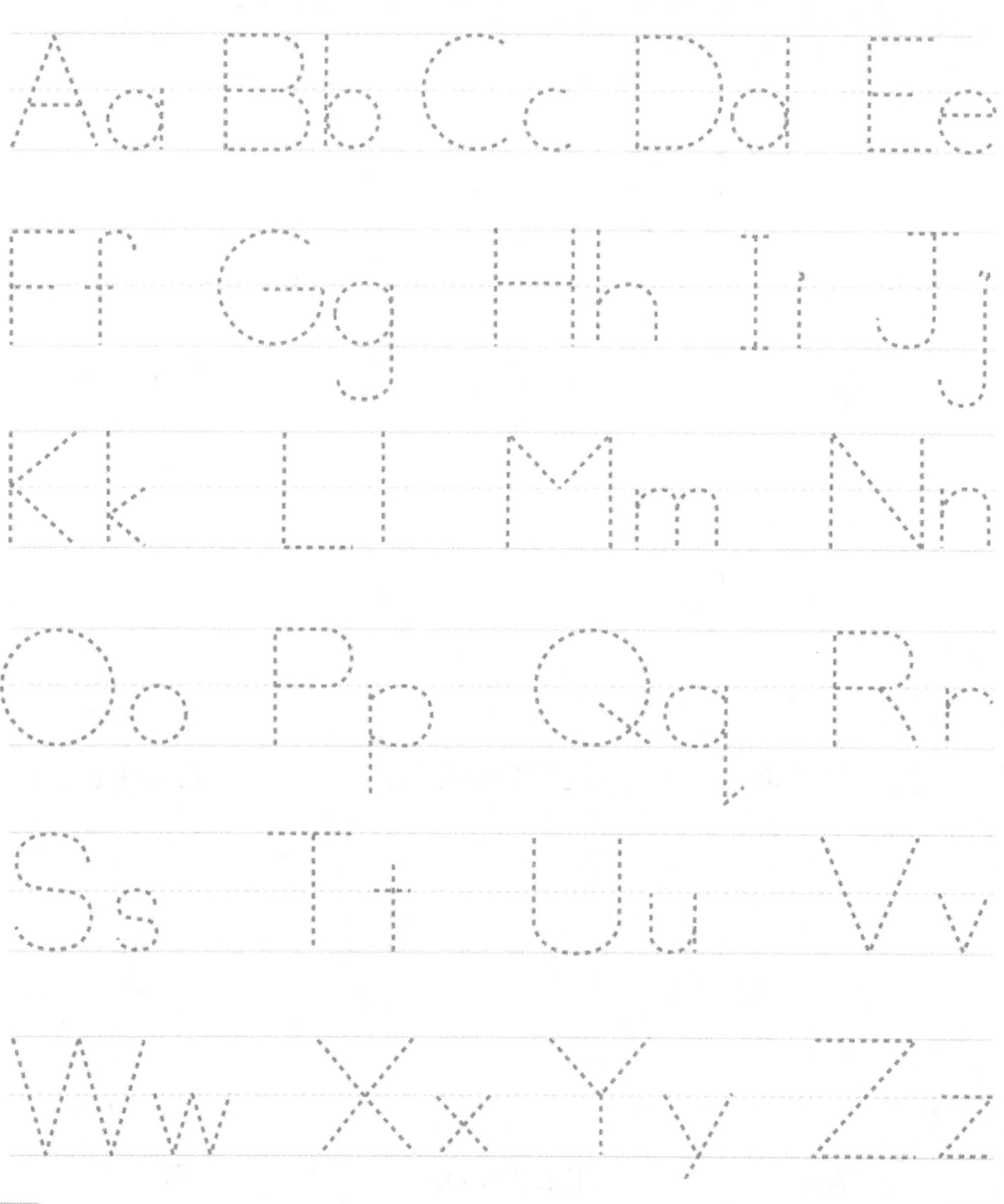

Trace the letters

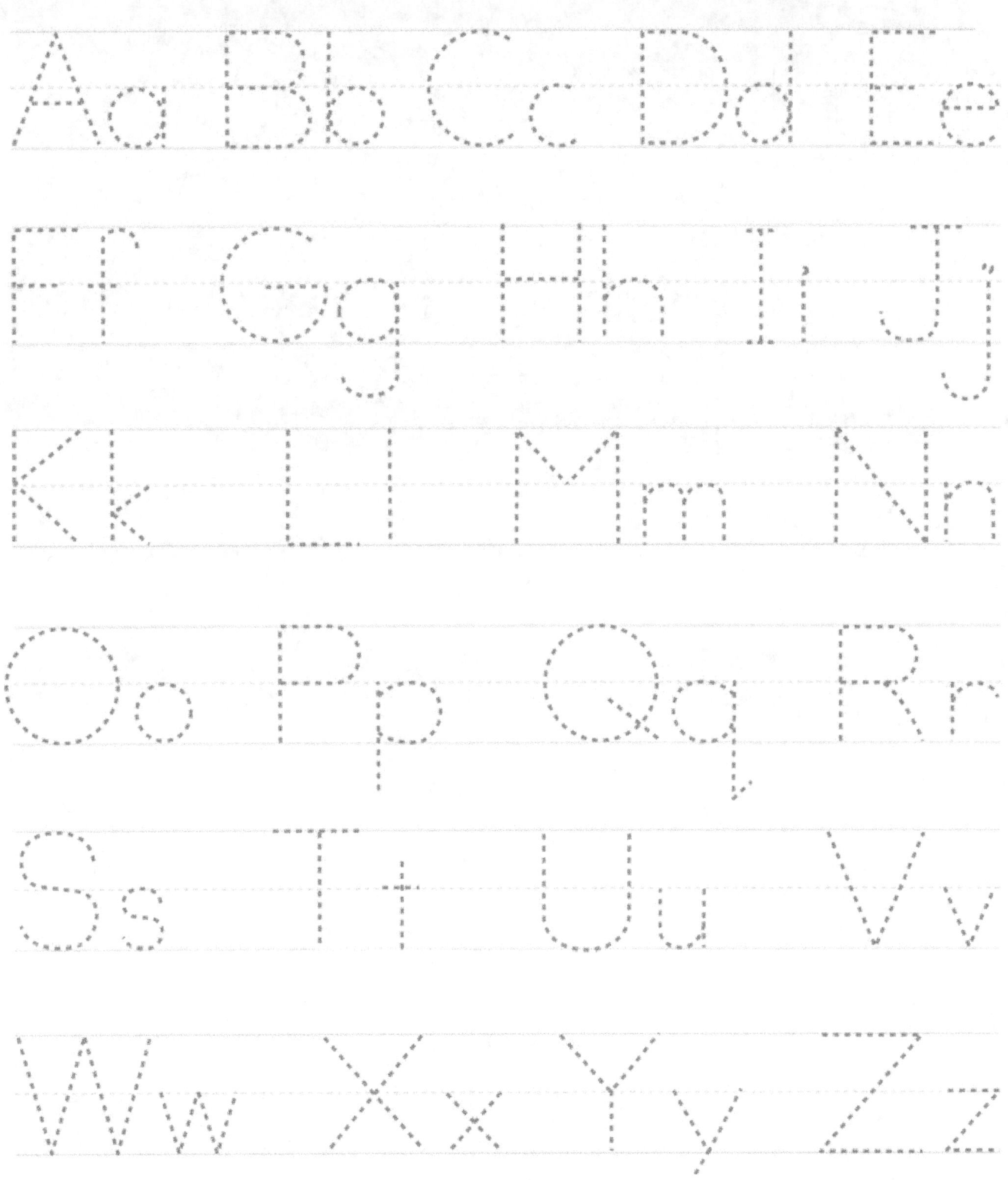

Trace the letters

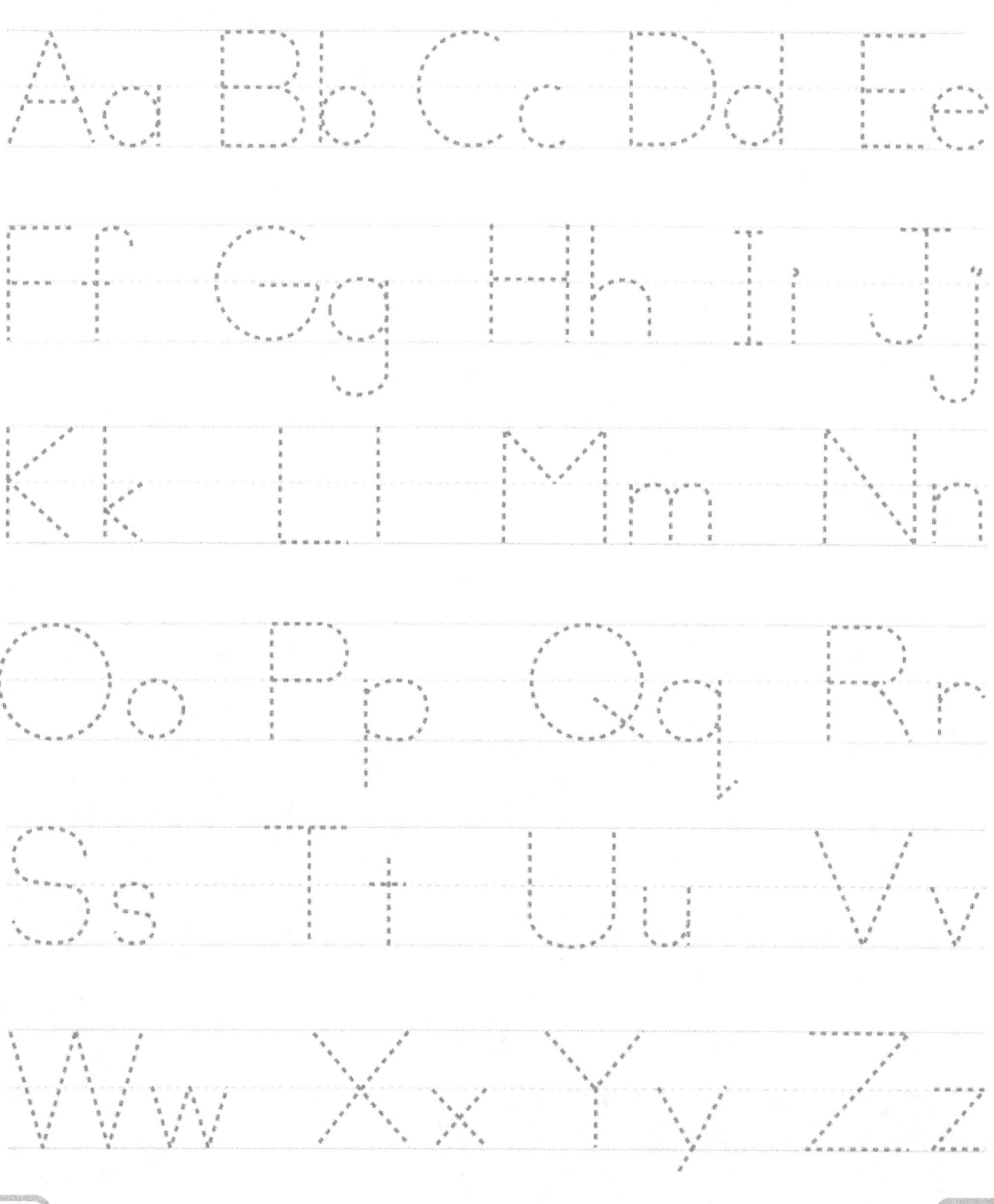

Trace the numbers

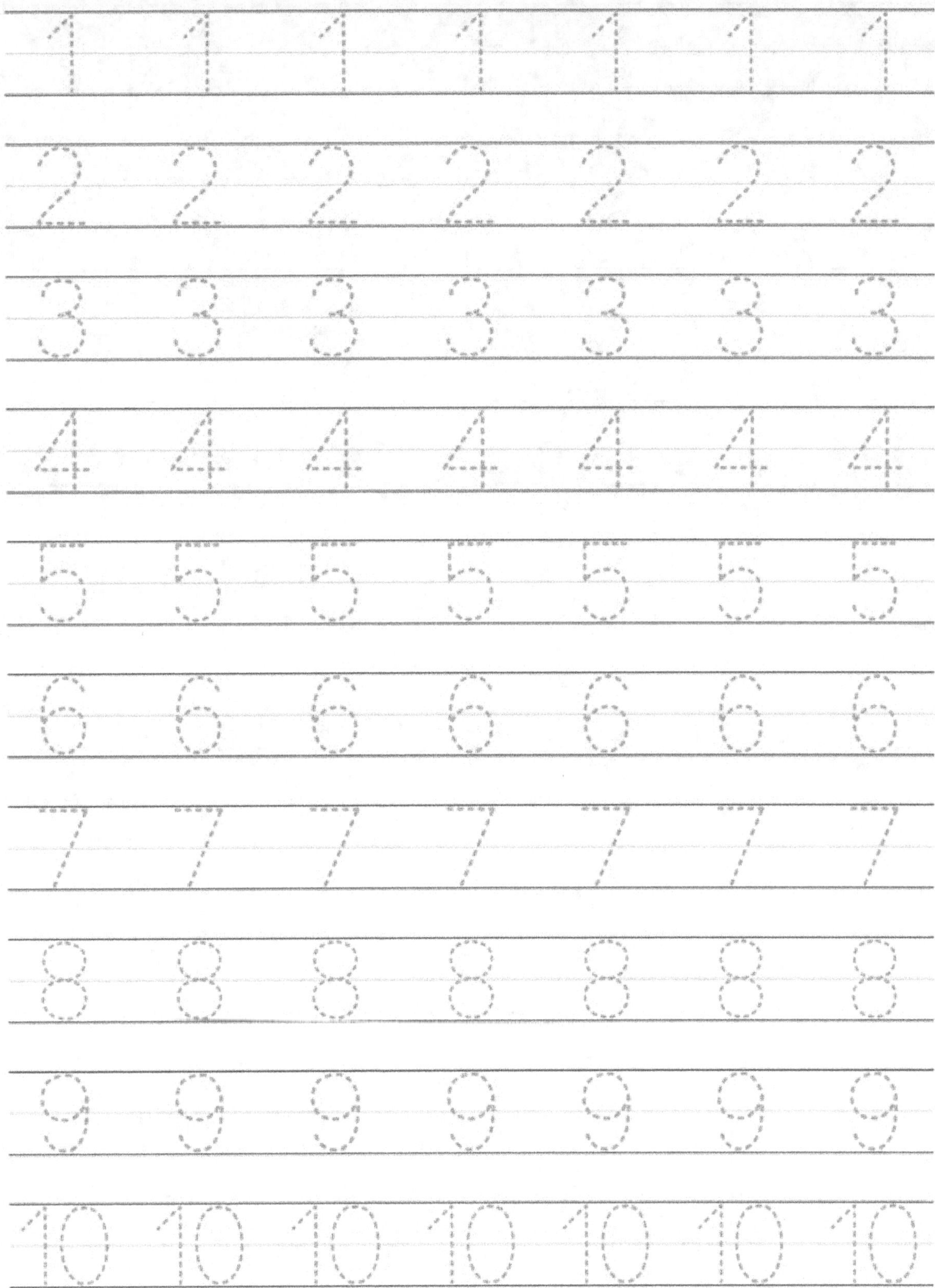

Trace the numbers

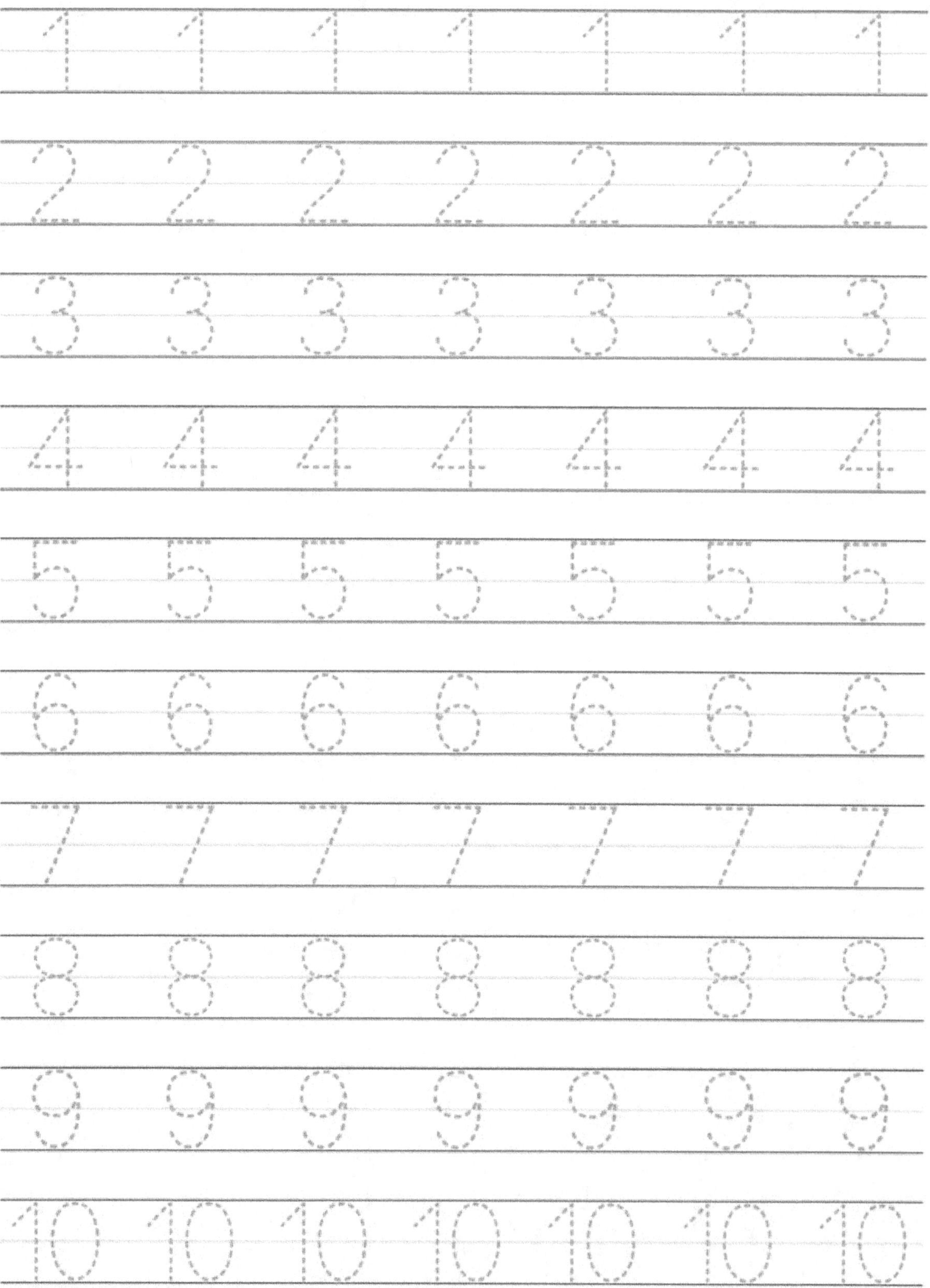

Trace the numbers

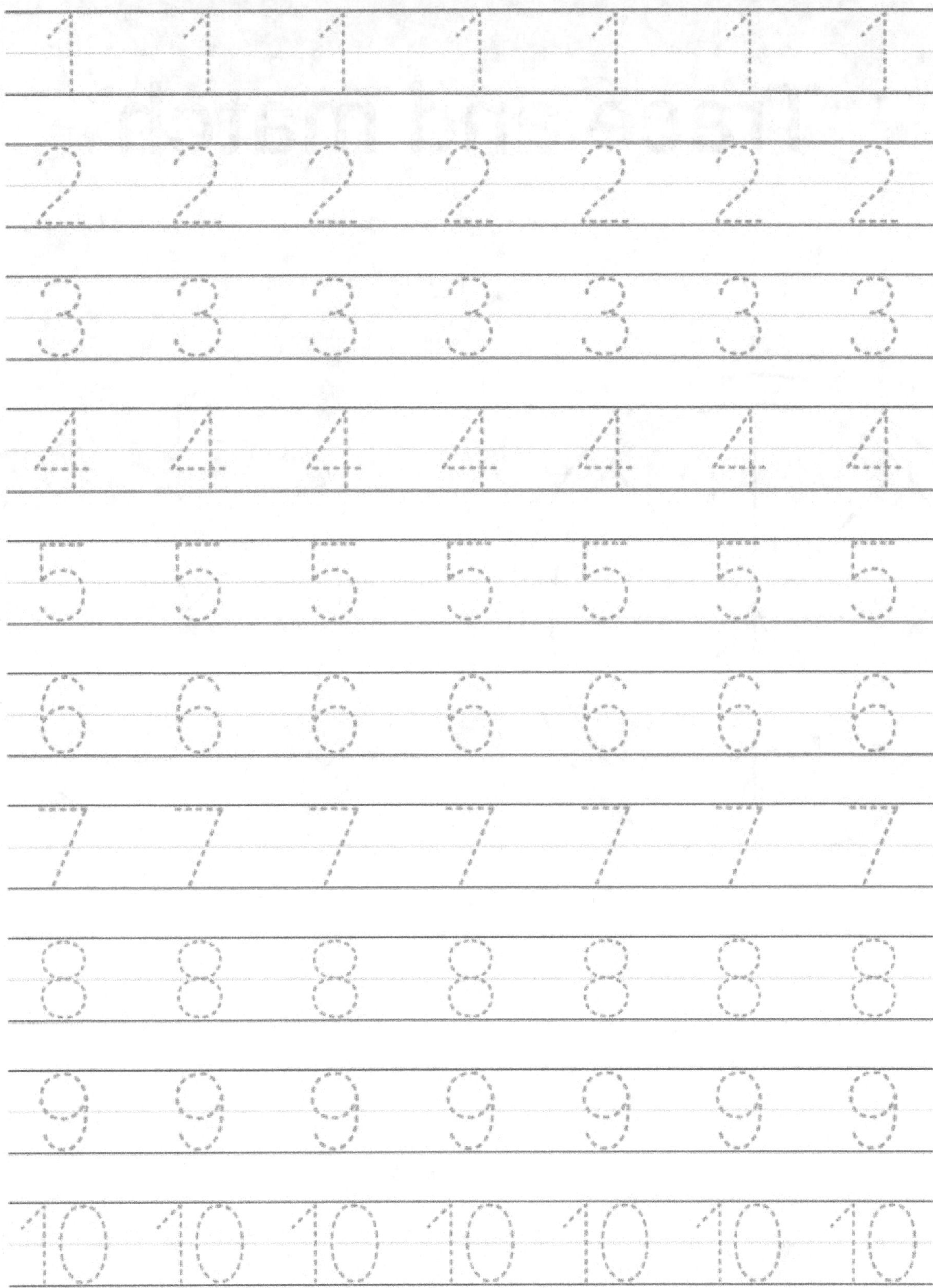

Trace and match

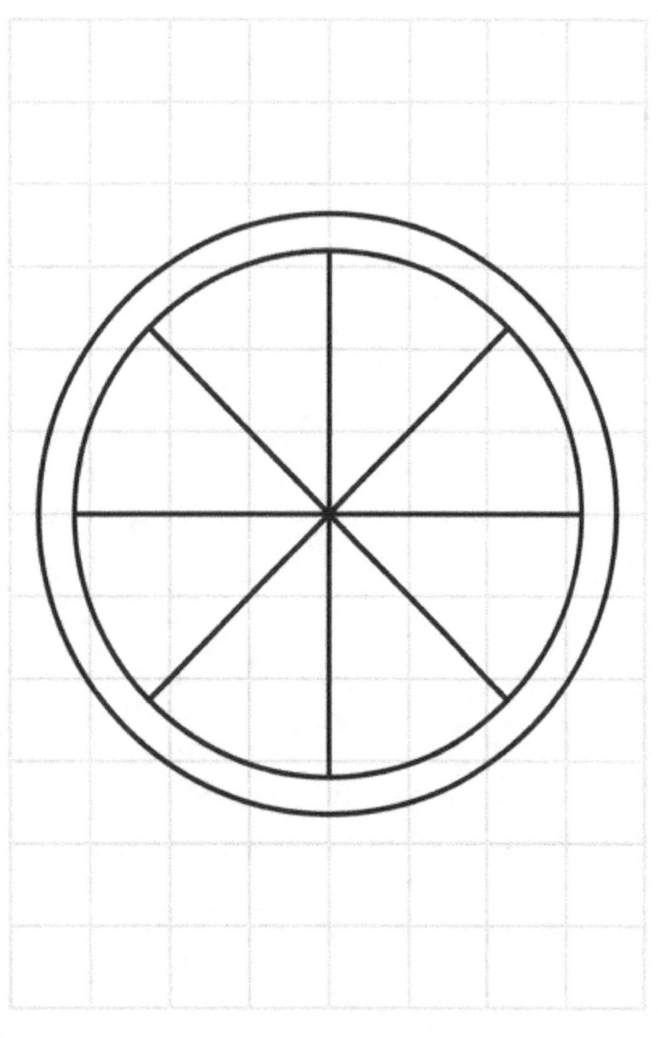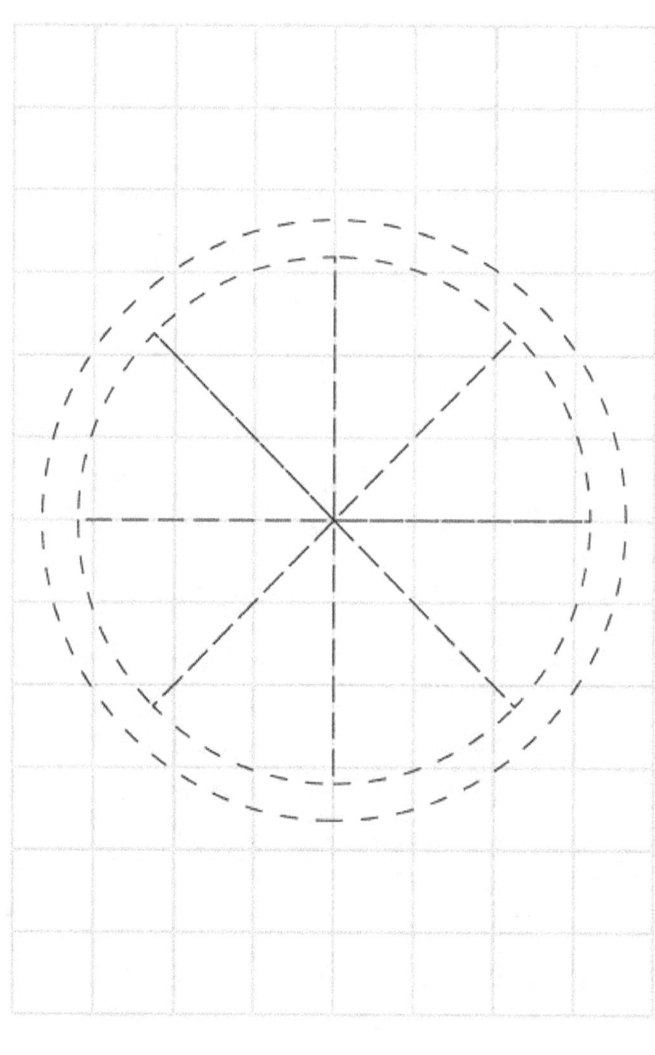

Trace and match

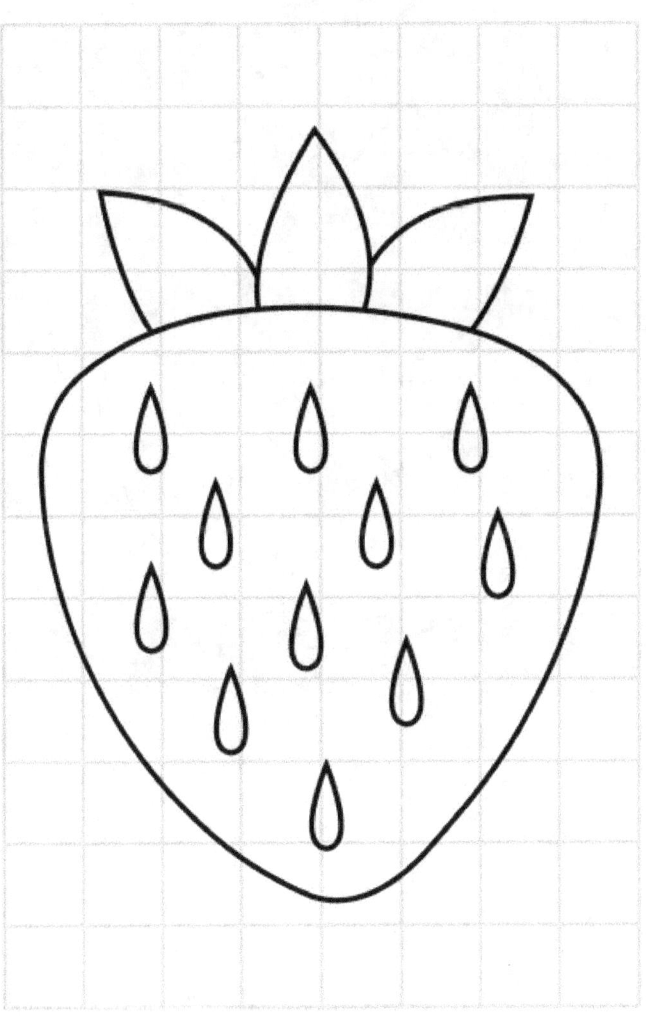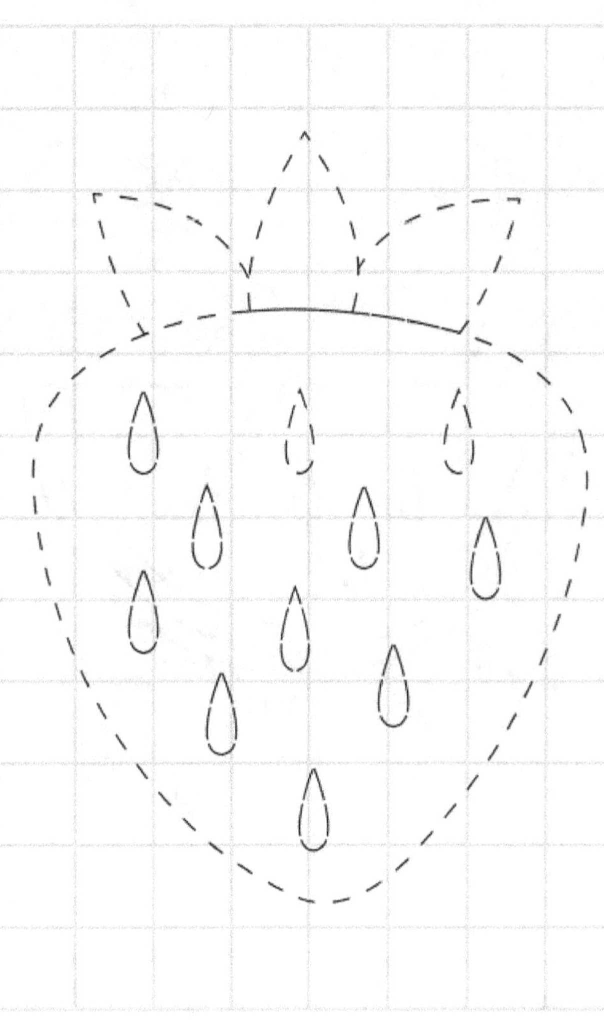

Trace and match

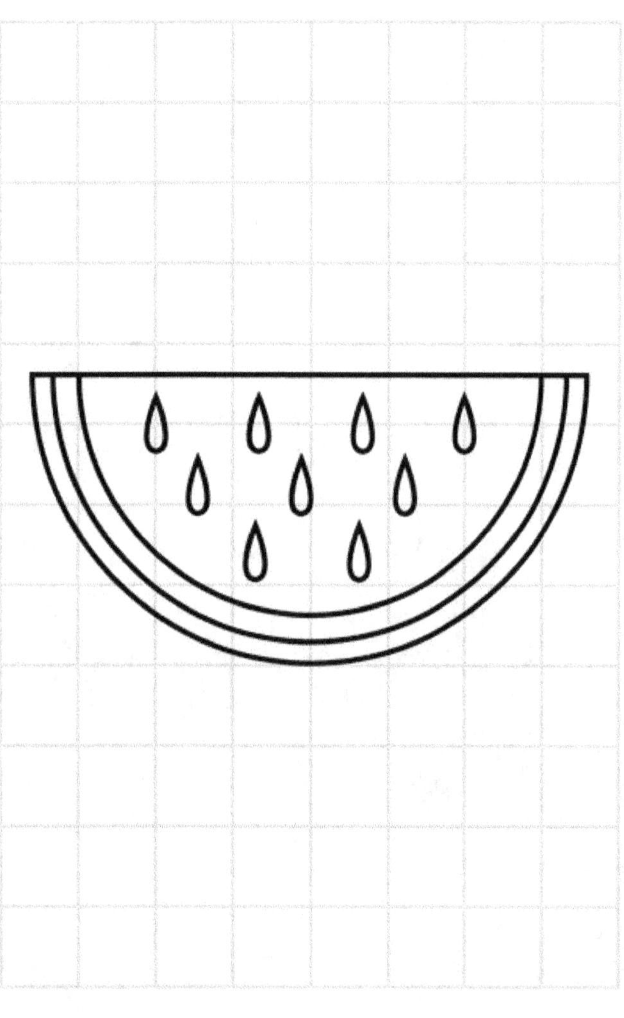 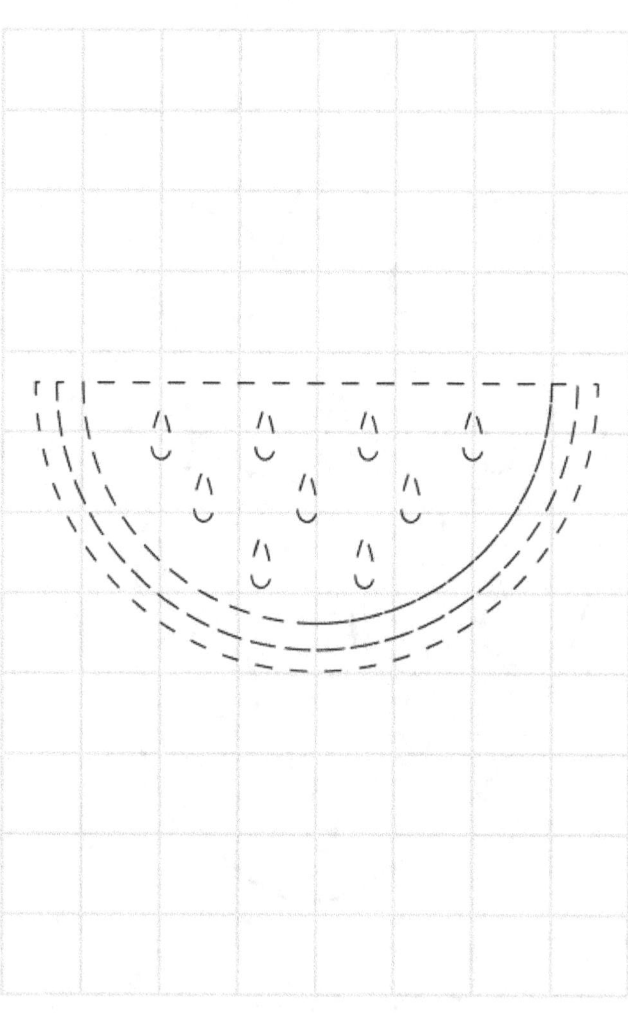

Connect the dots

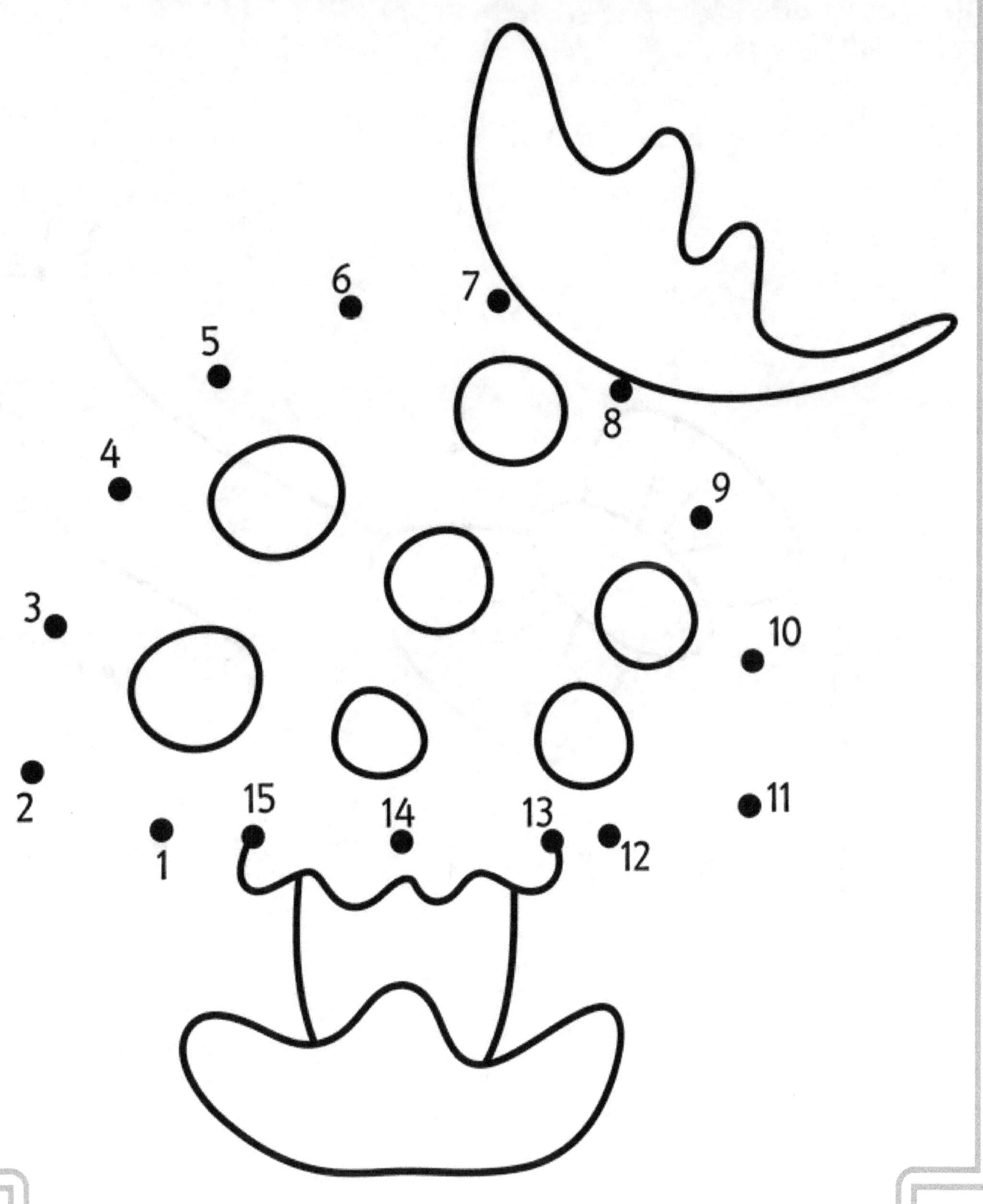

Connect the dots

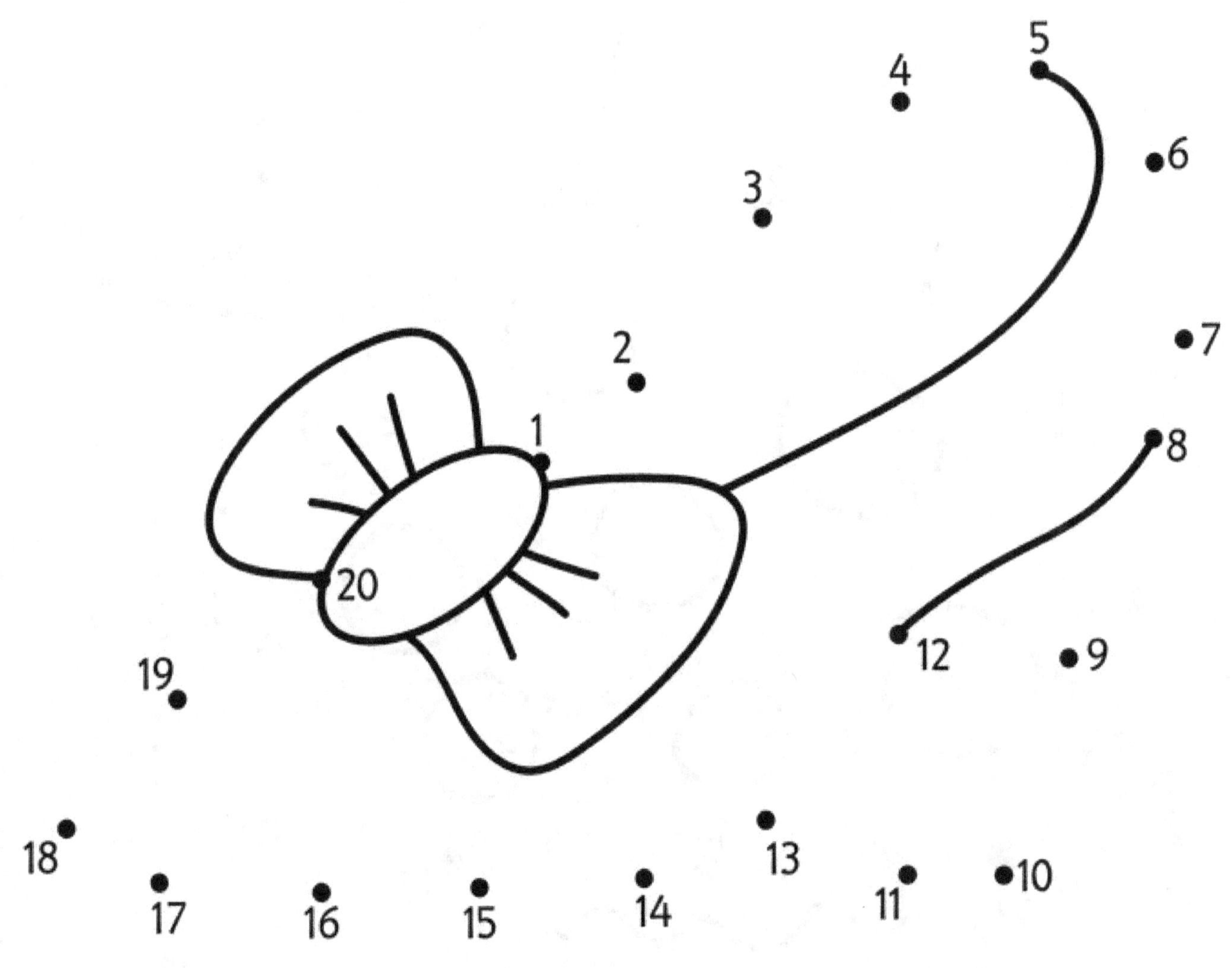

Connect the dots

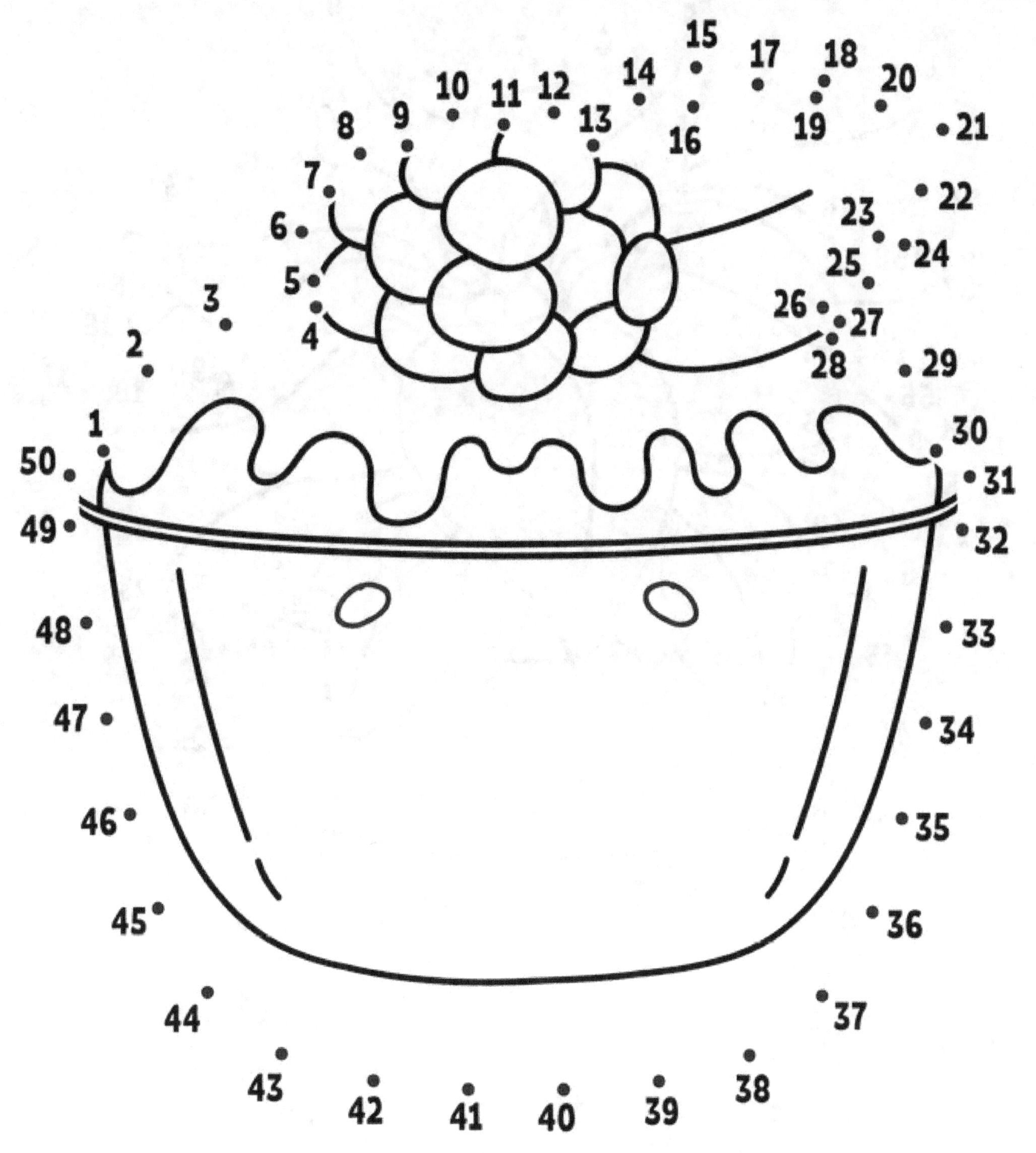

Connect the dots

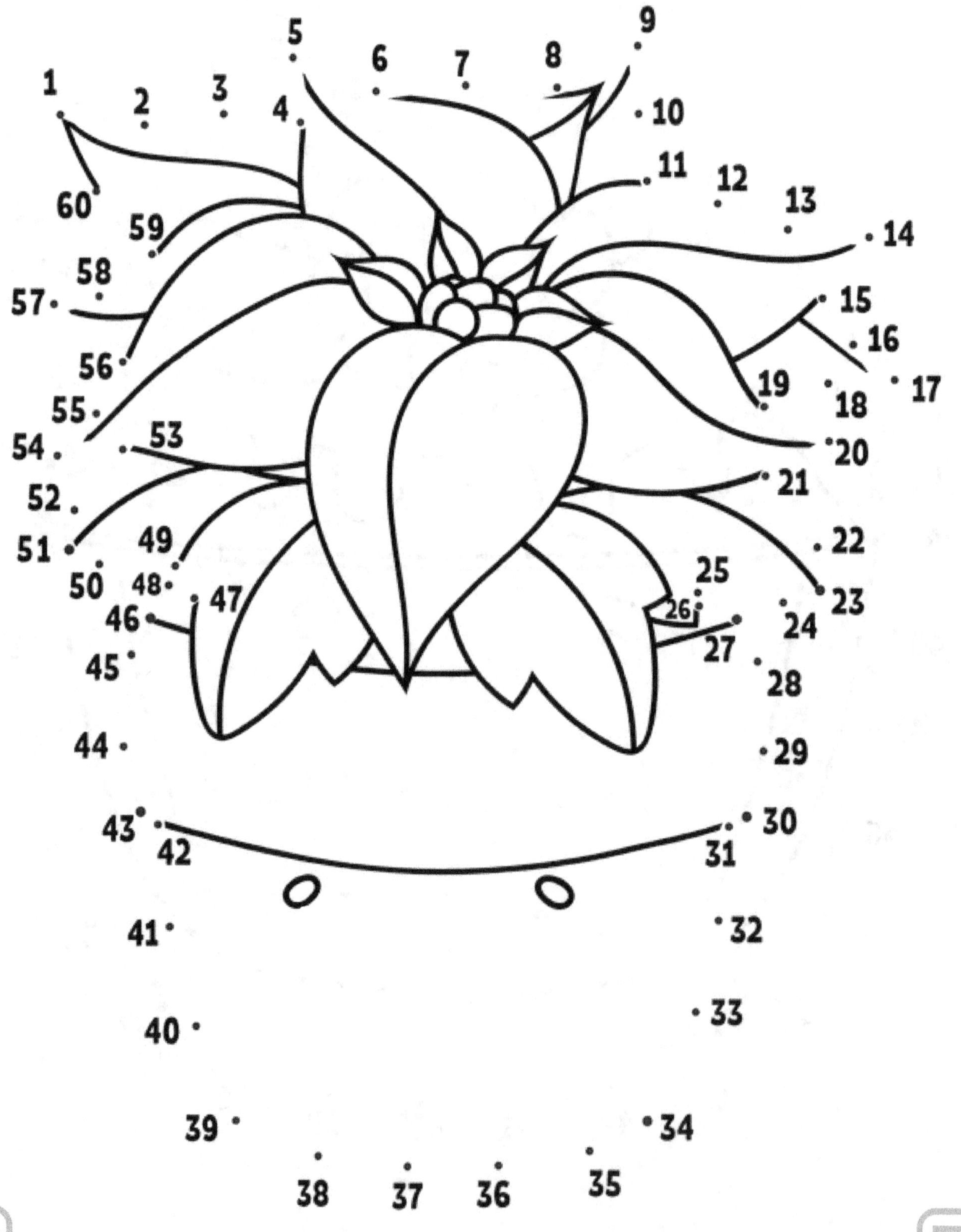

Symmetry drawing

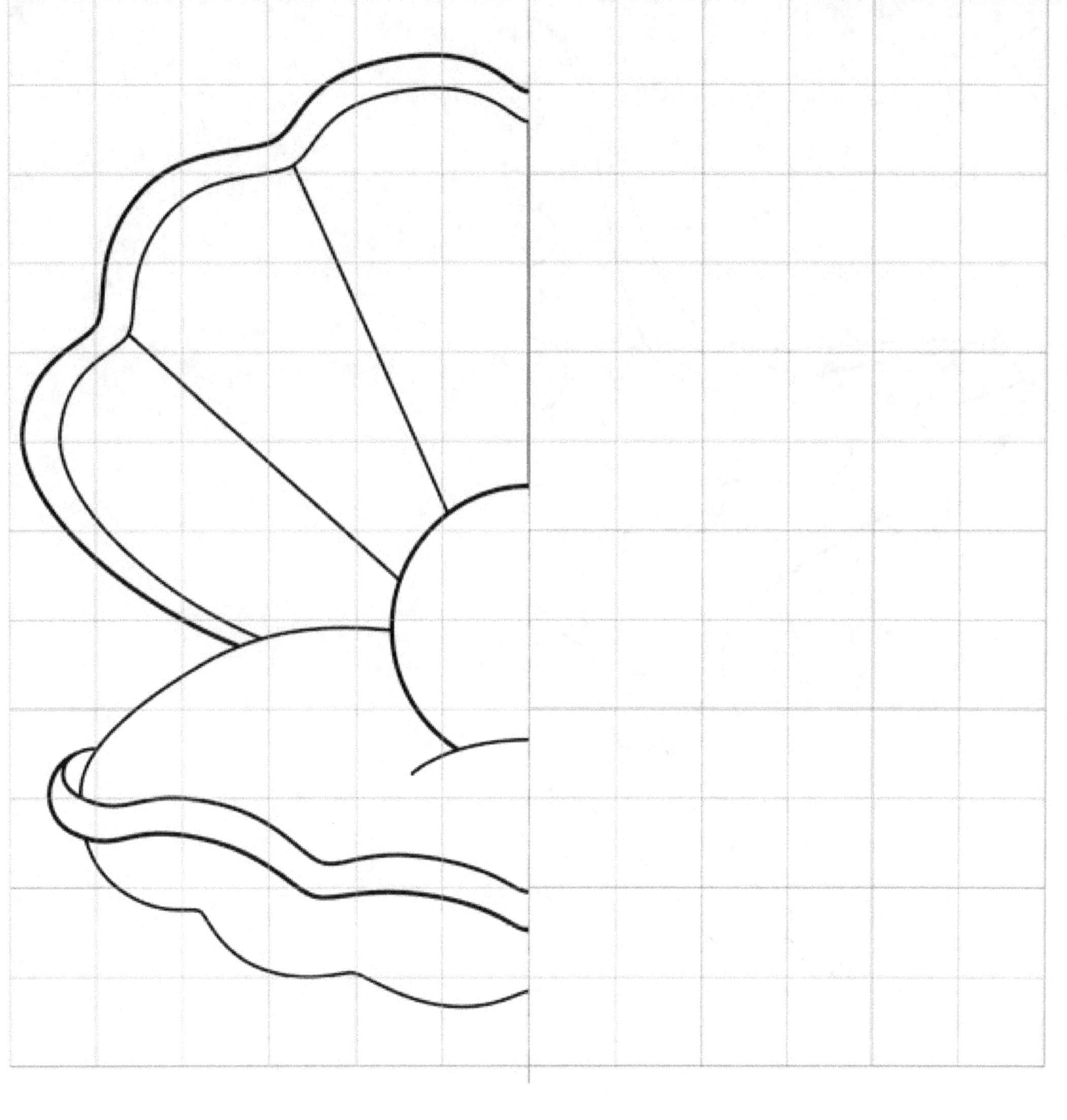

Symmetry drawing

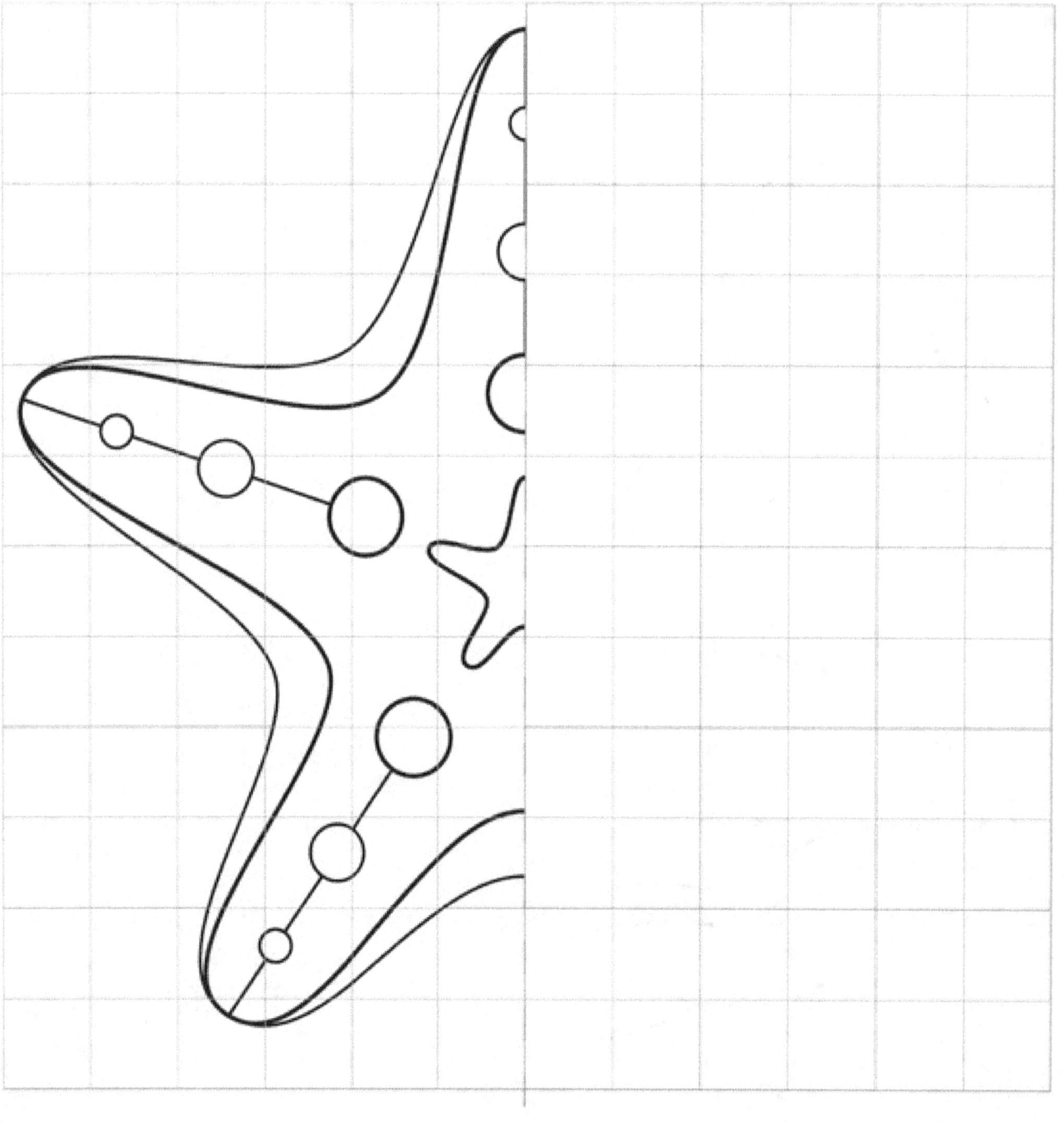

Symmetry drawing

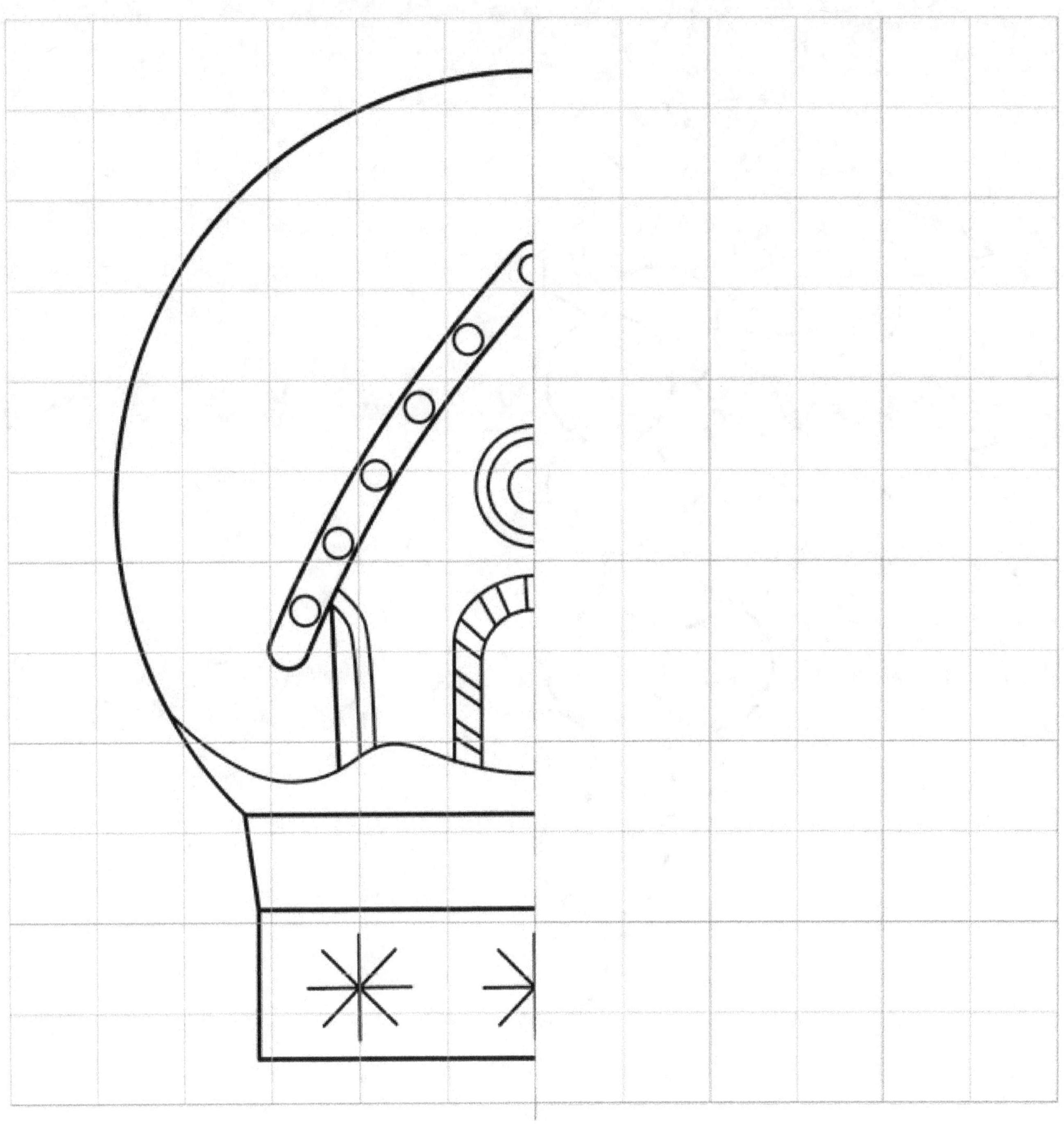

Symmetry drawing

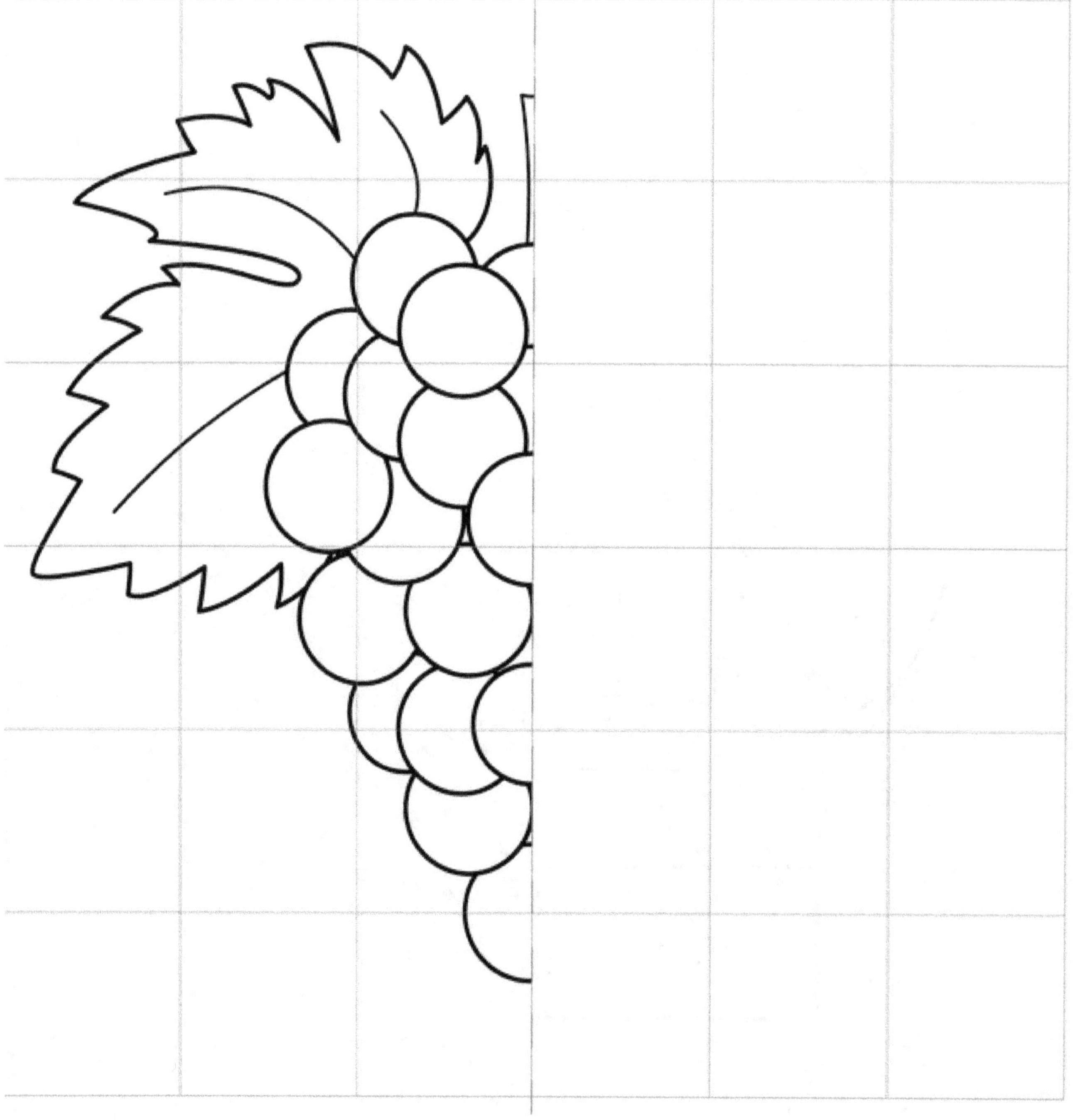

Shadow matching

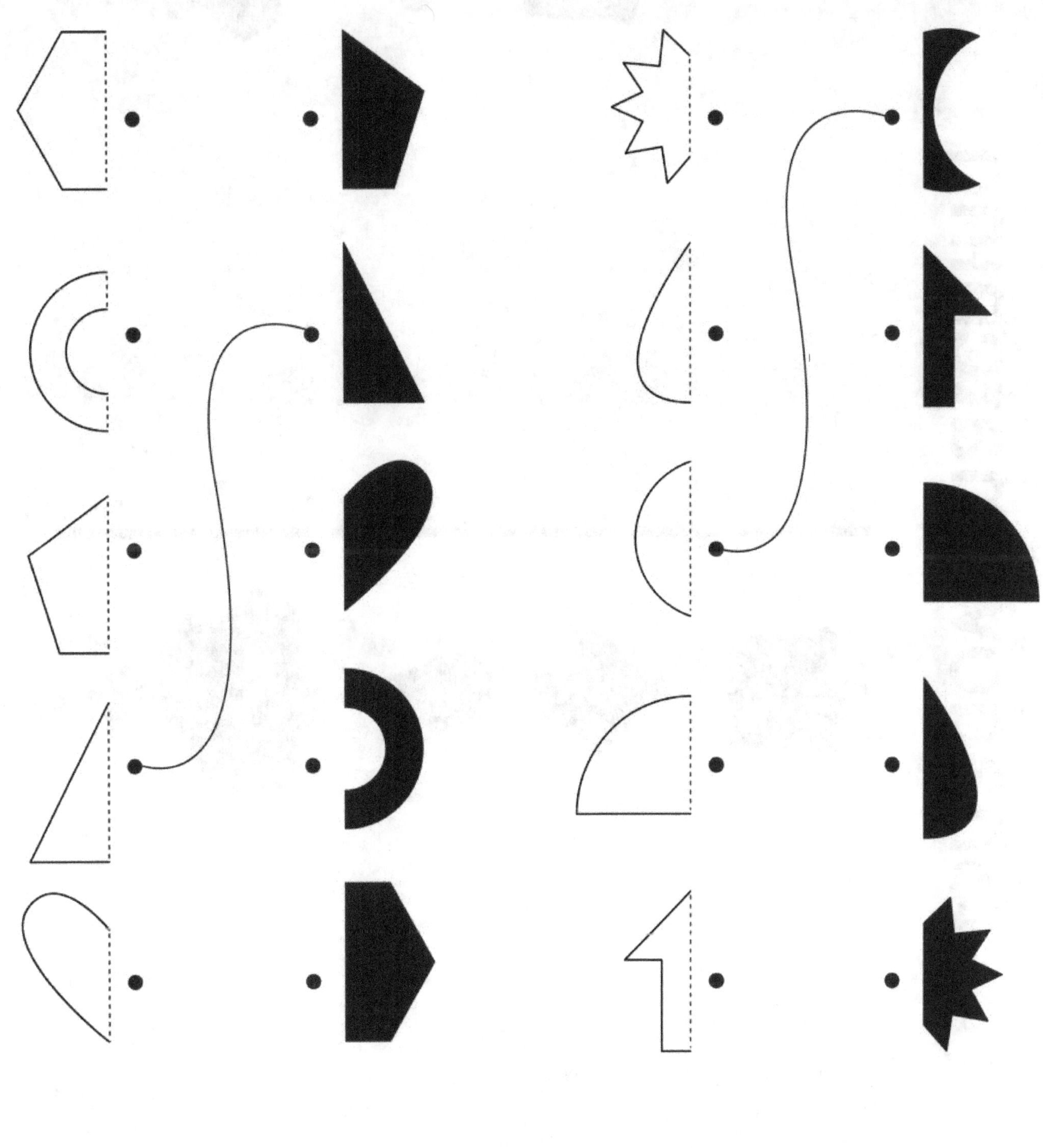

Shadow matching

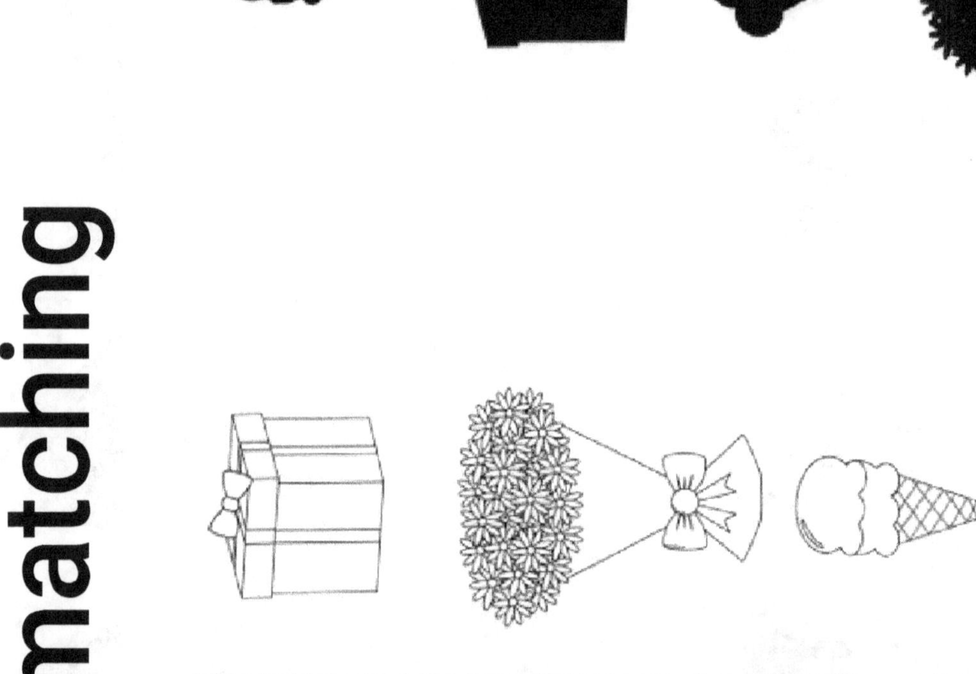

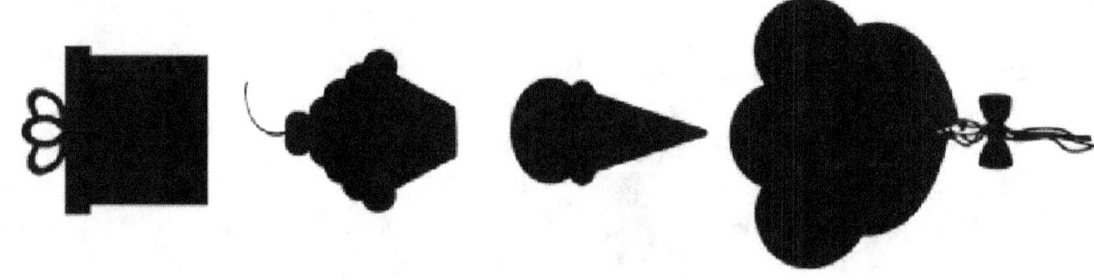

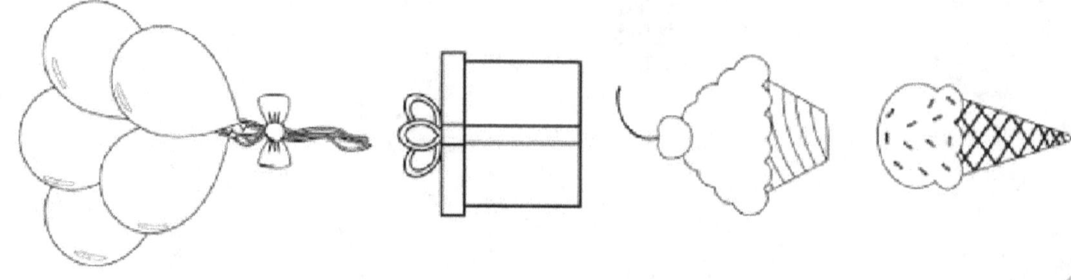

Shadow matching

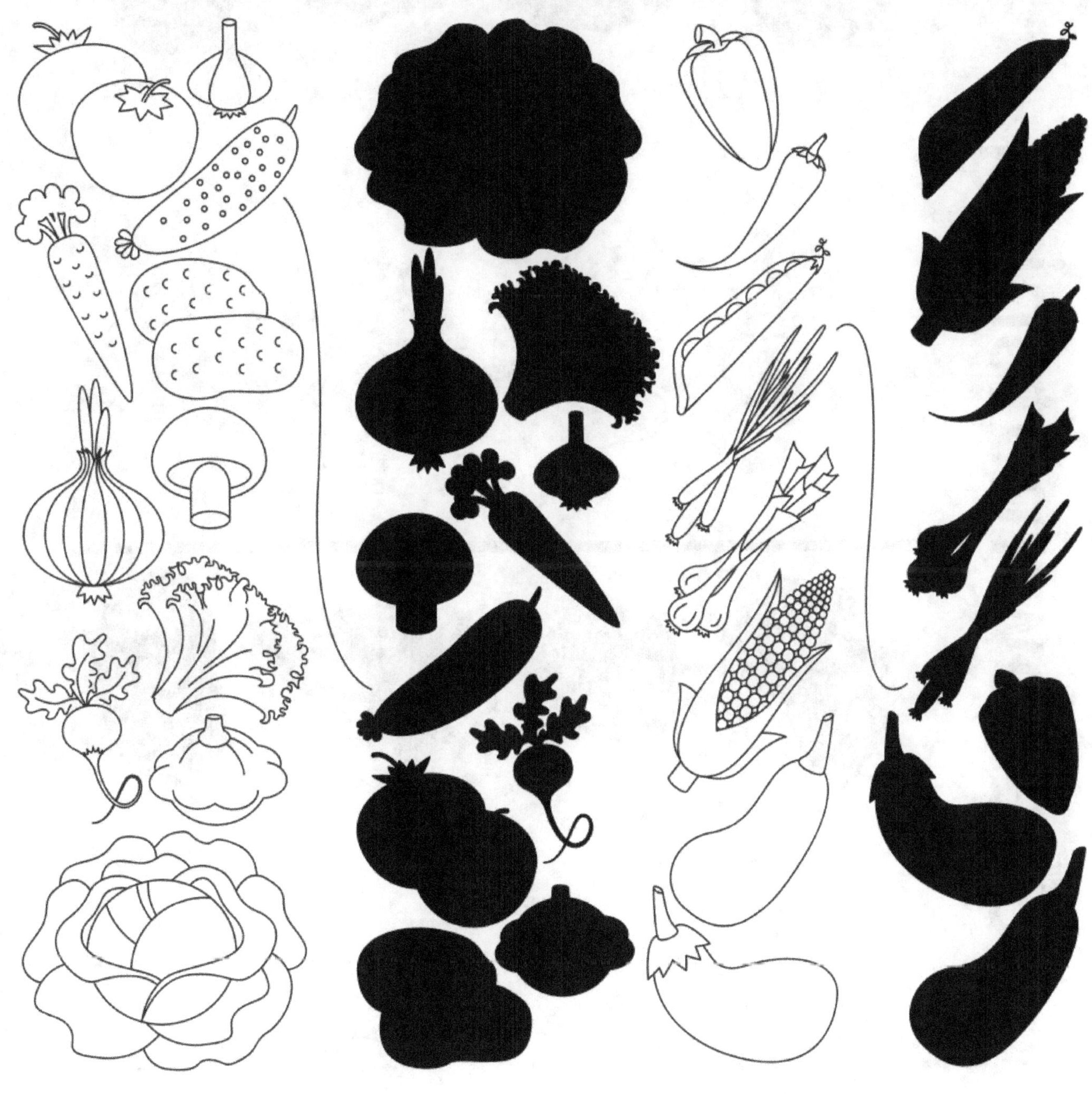

Shadow matching

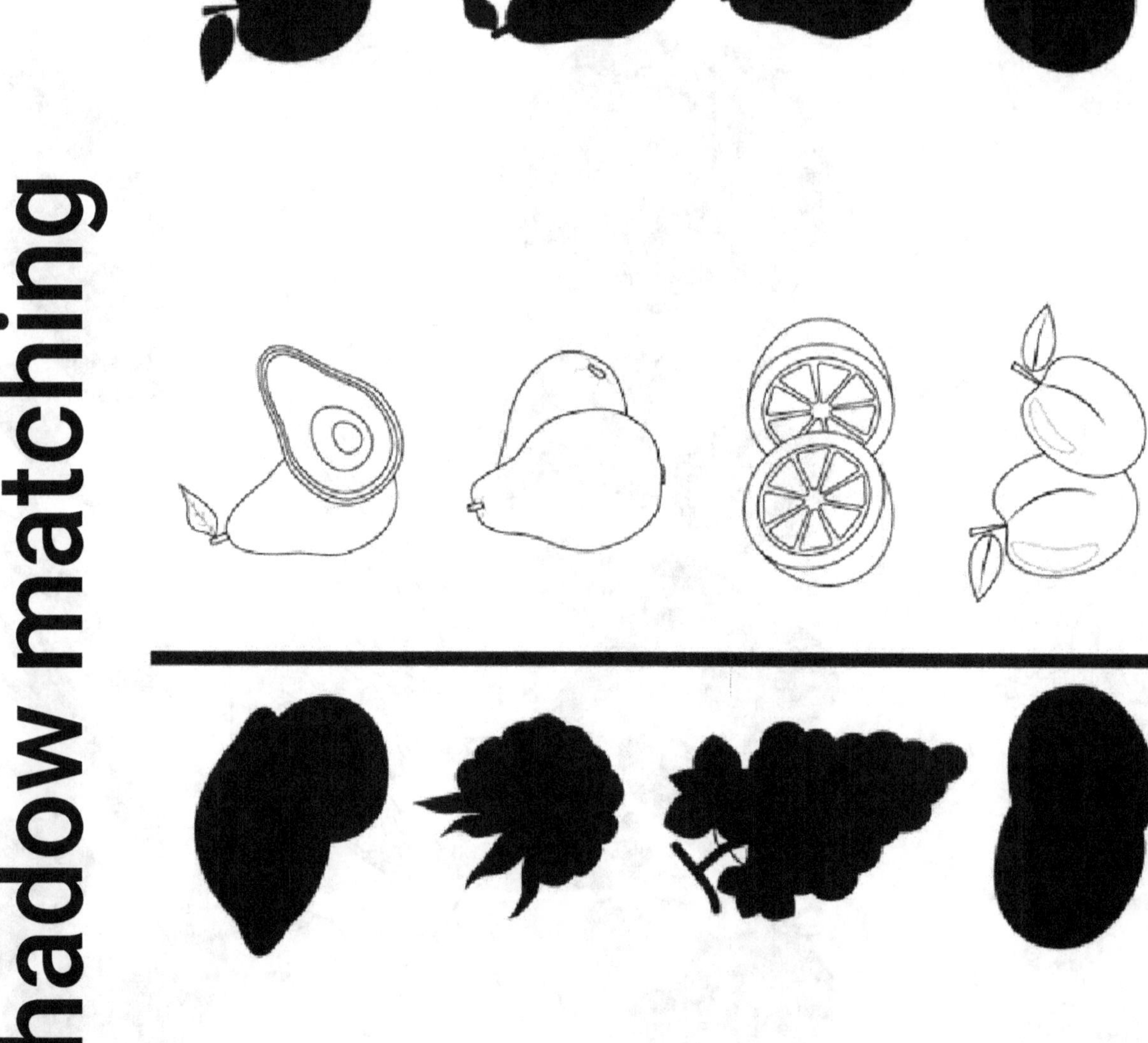

Item hunt

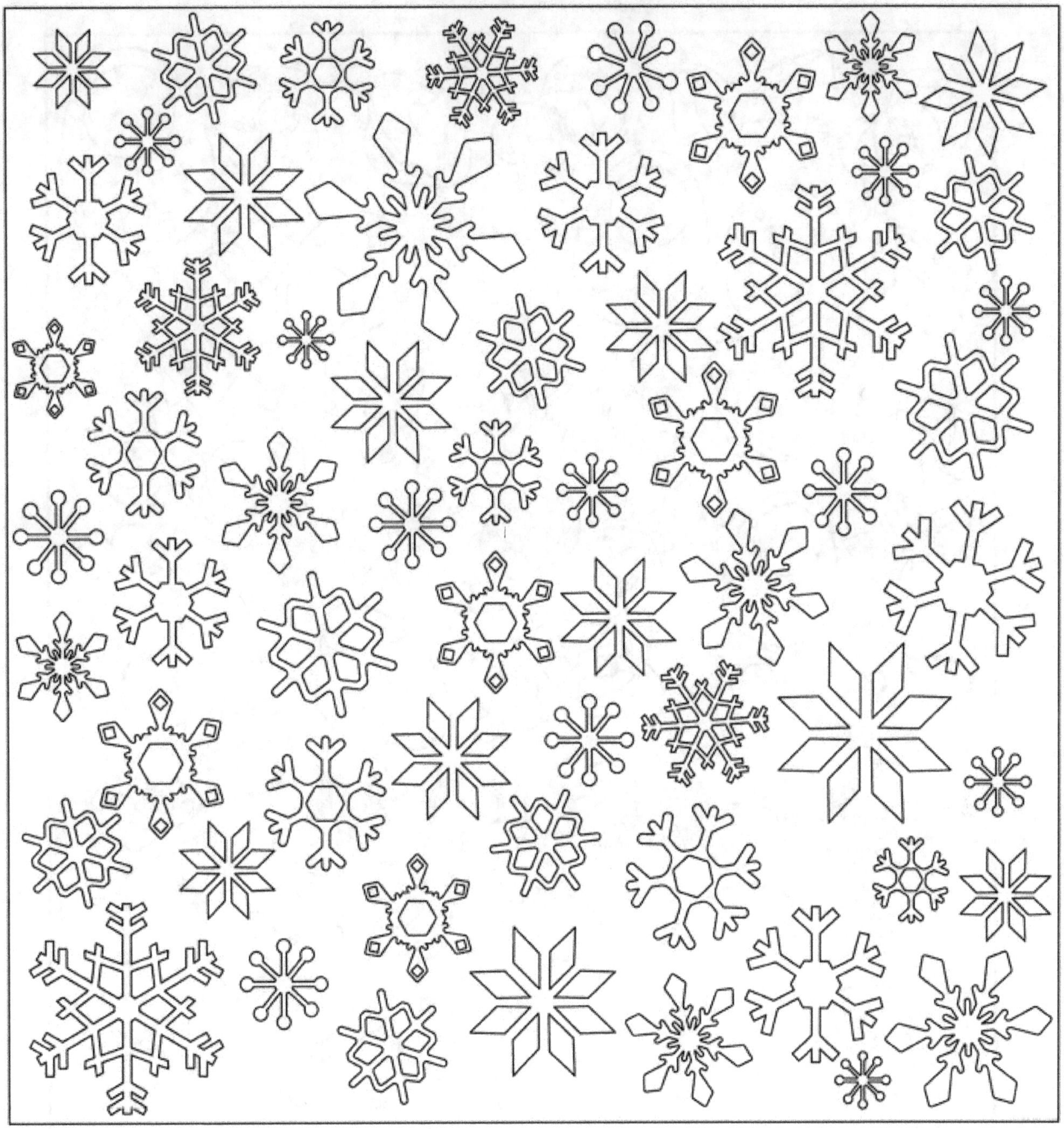

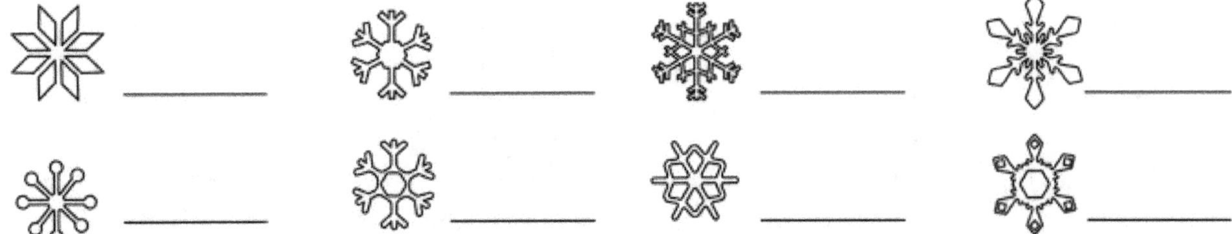

Item hunt

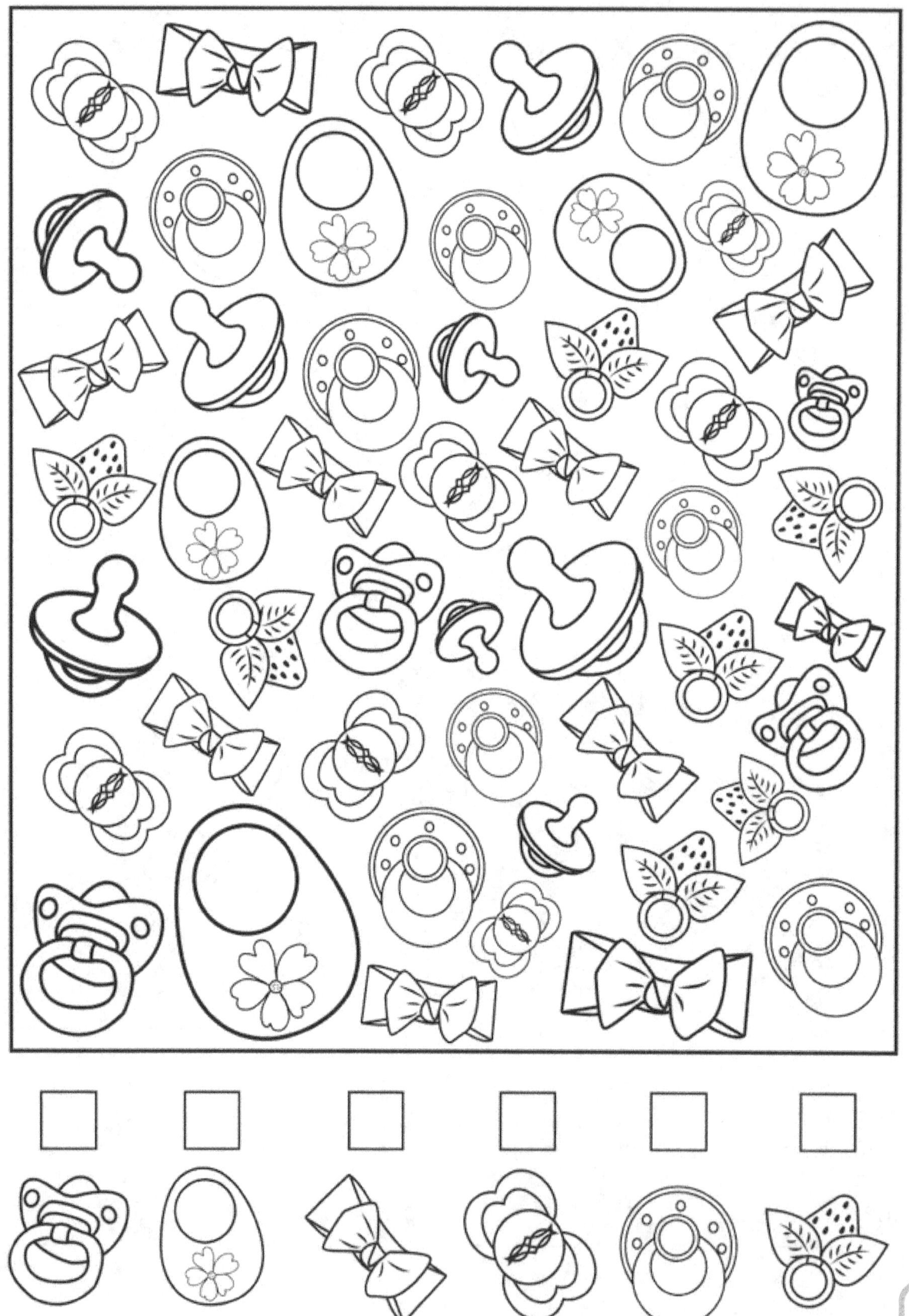

Item hunt

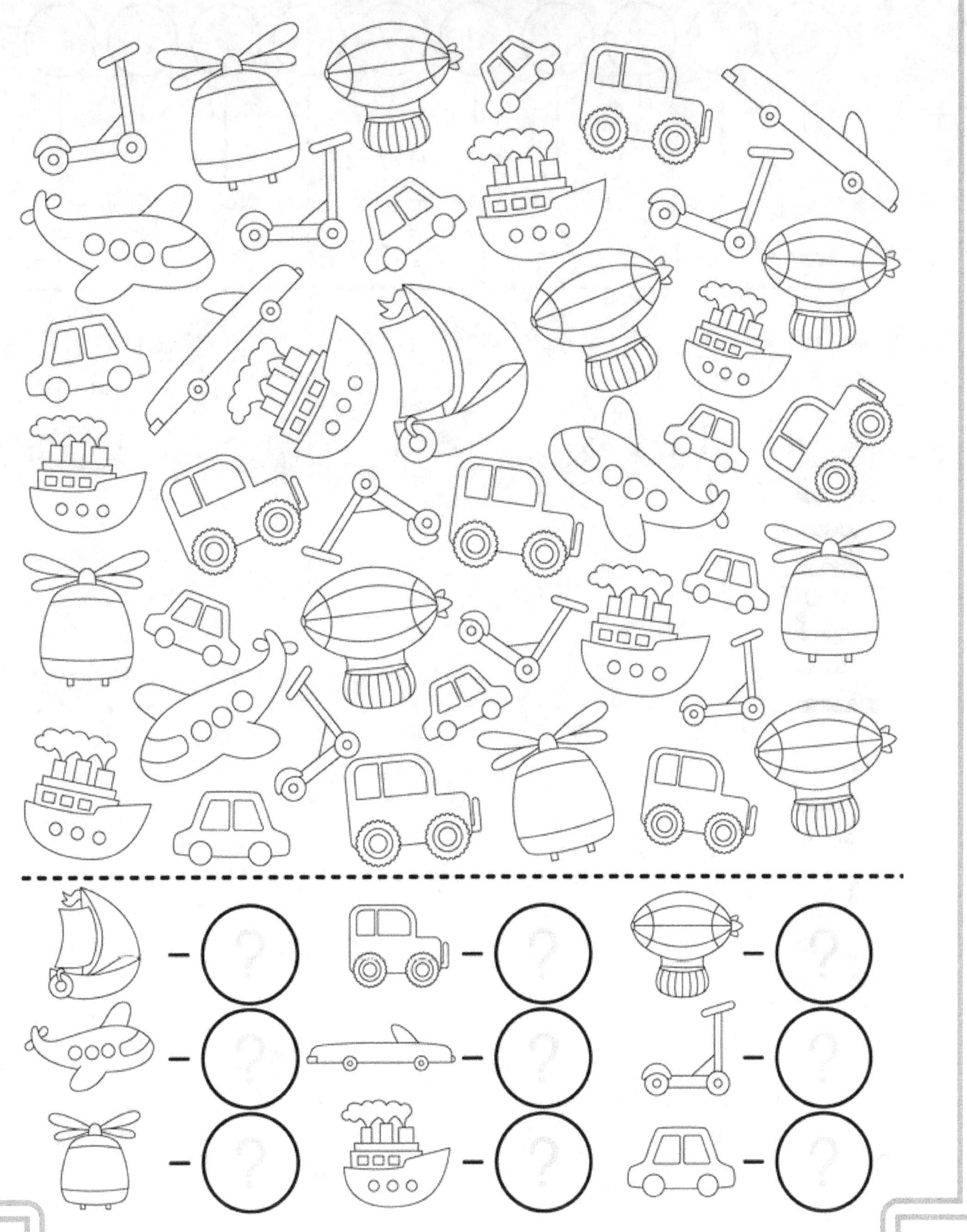

Item hunt

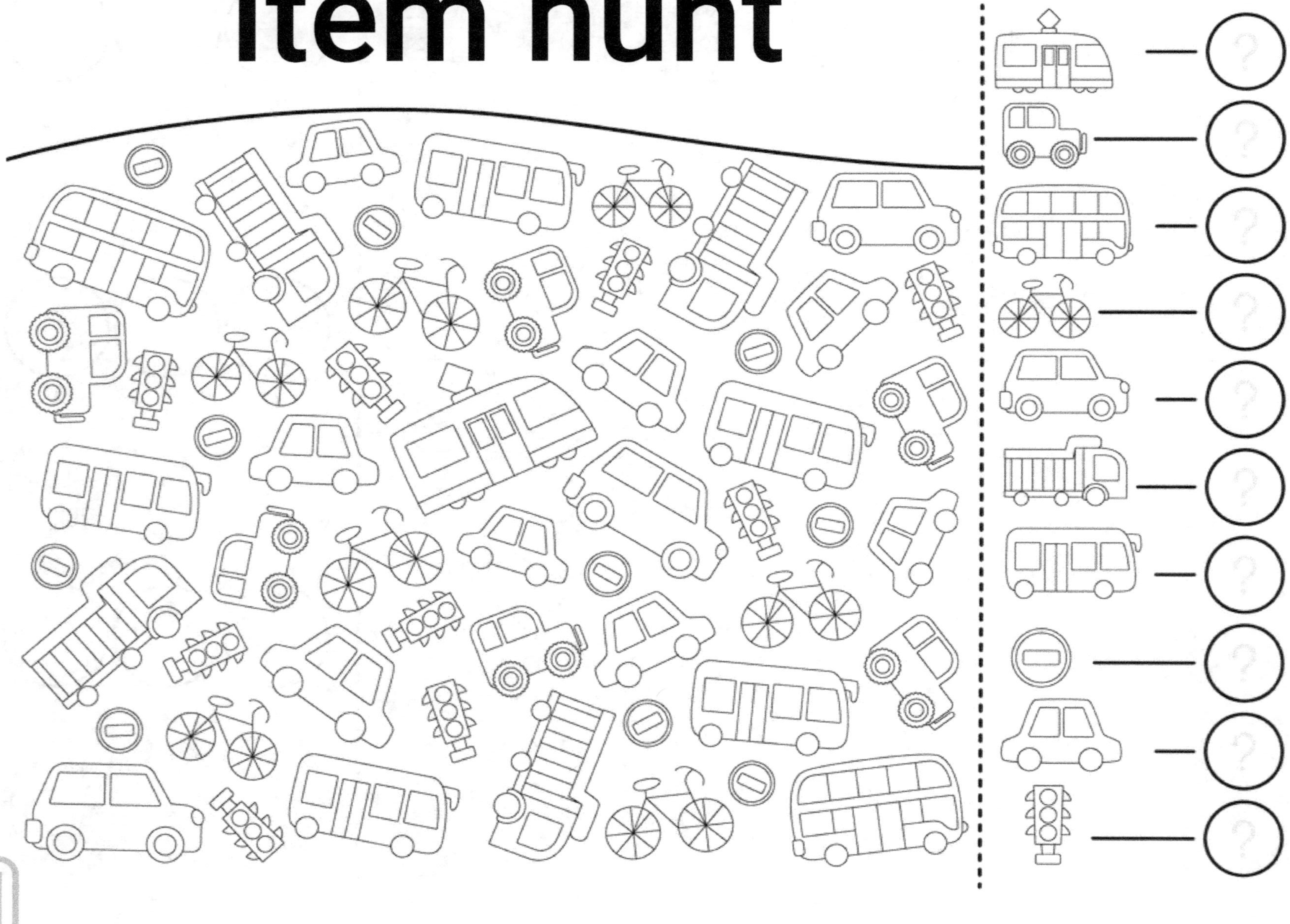

Item hunt

Coloring page

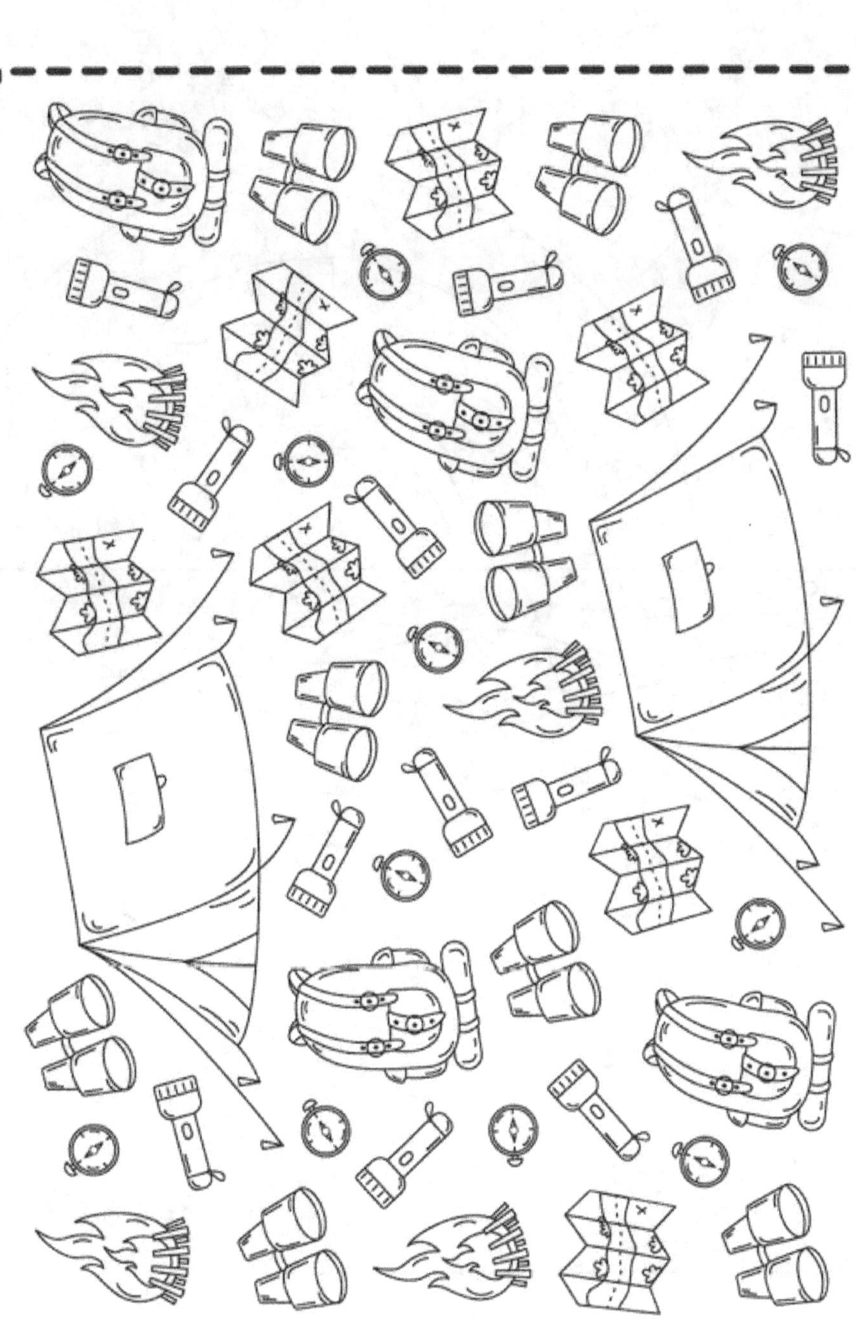

Coloring pages

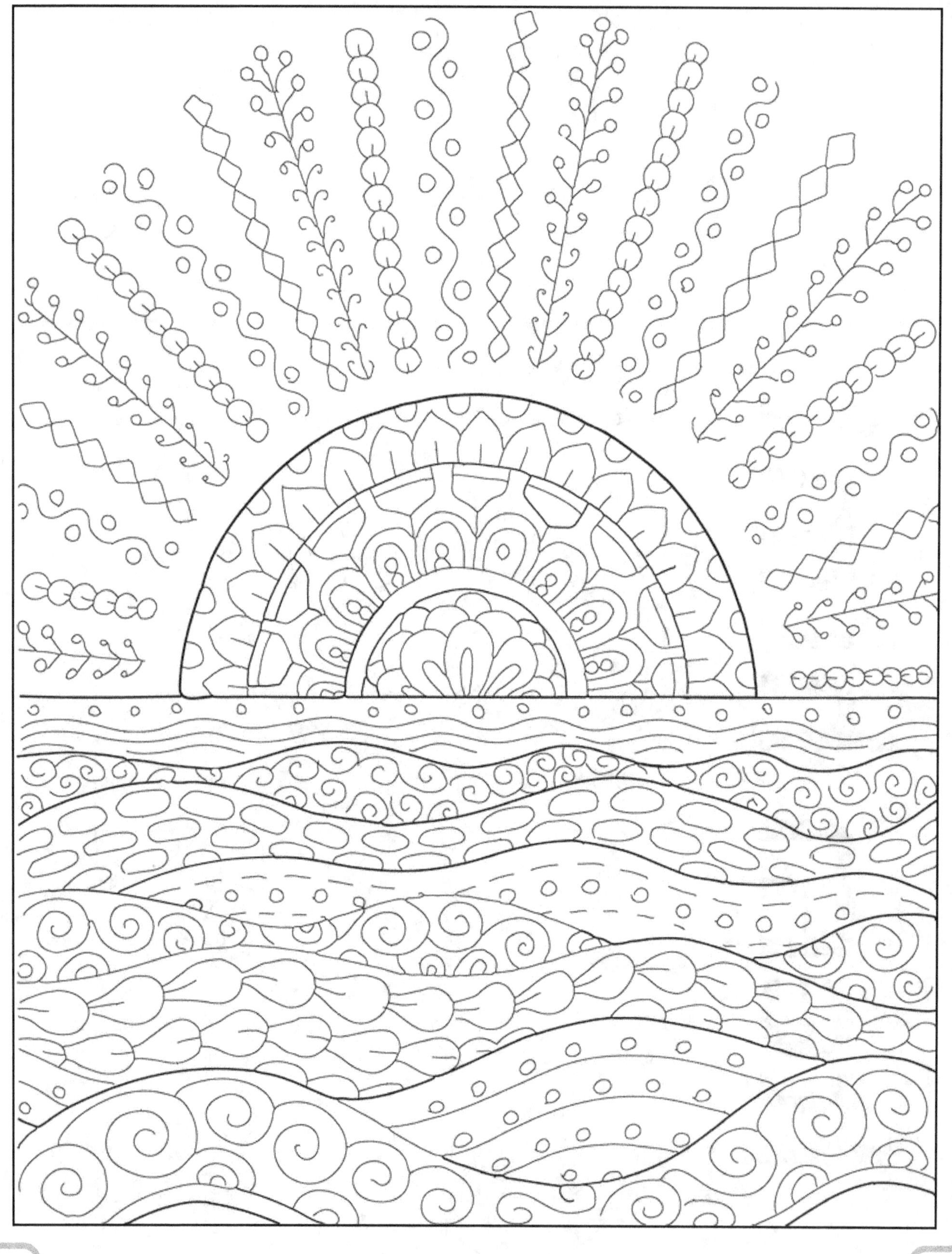

Coloring pages

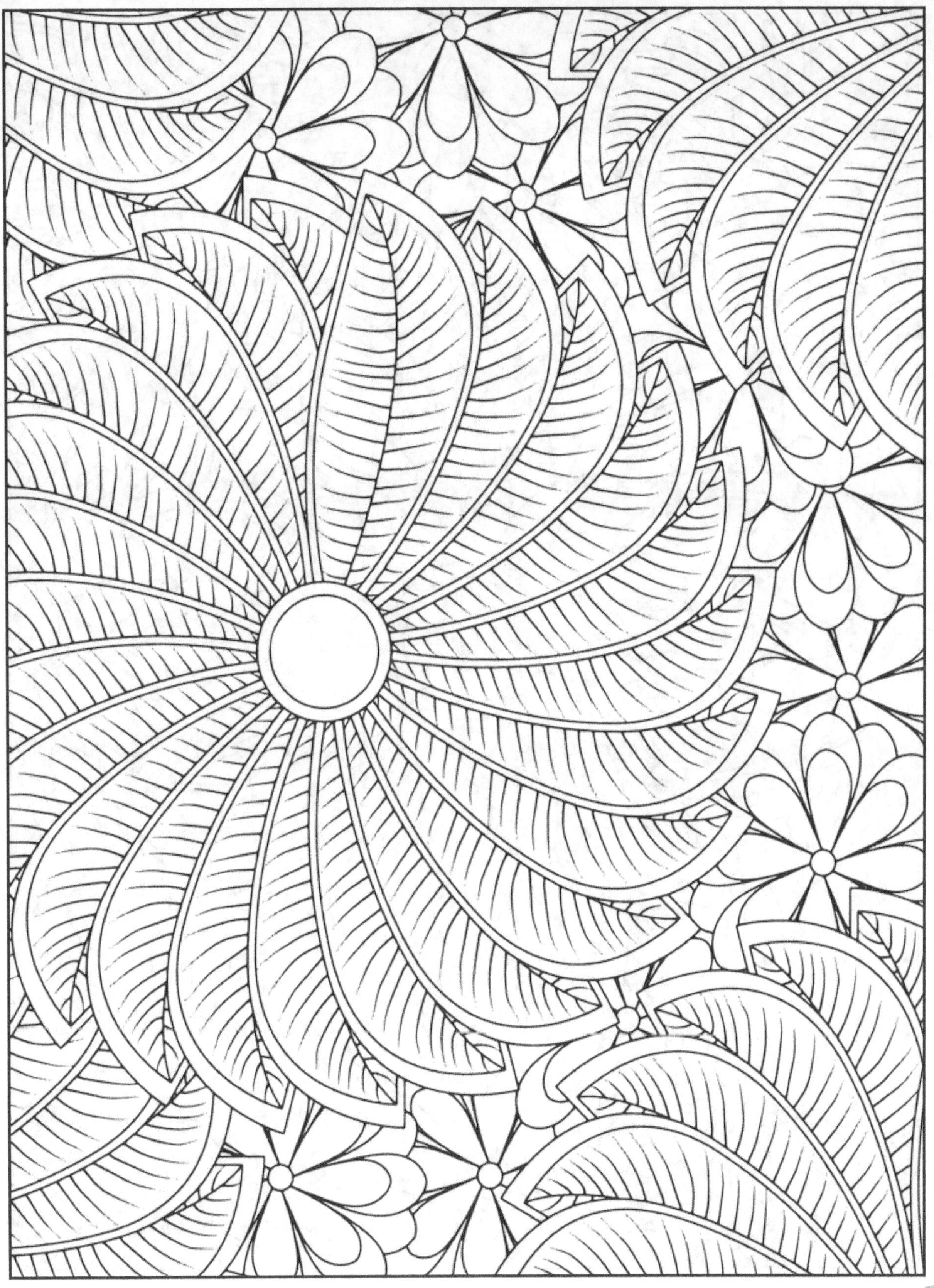

Coloring pages

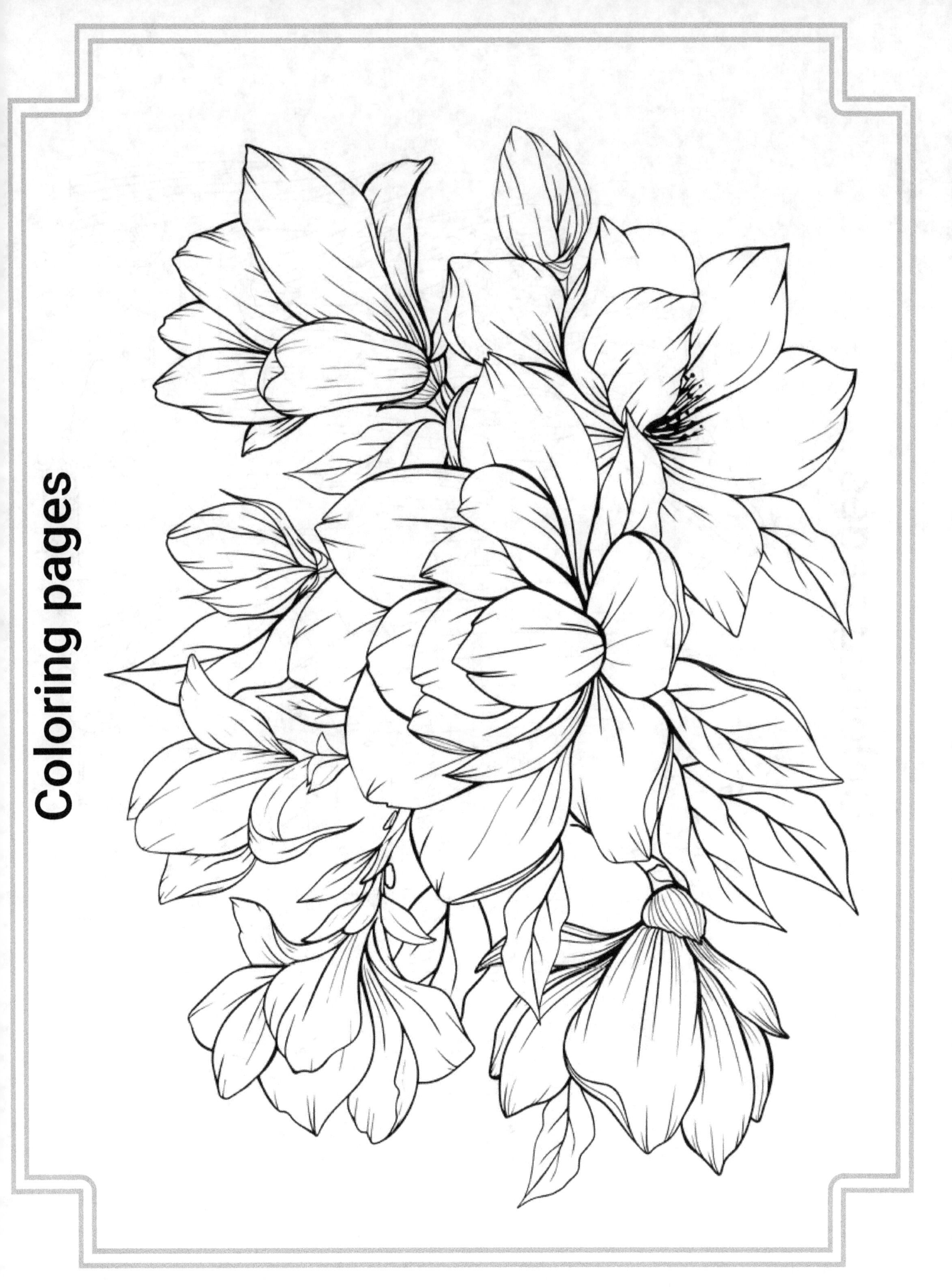
Coloring pages

Coloring pages

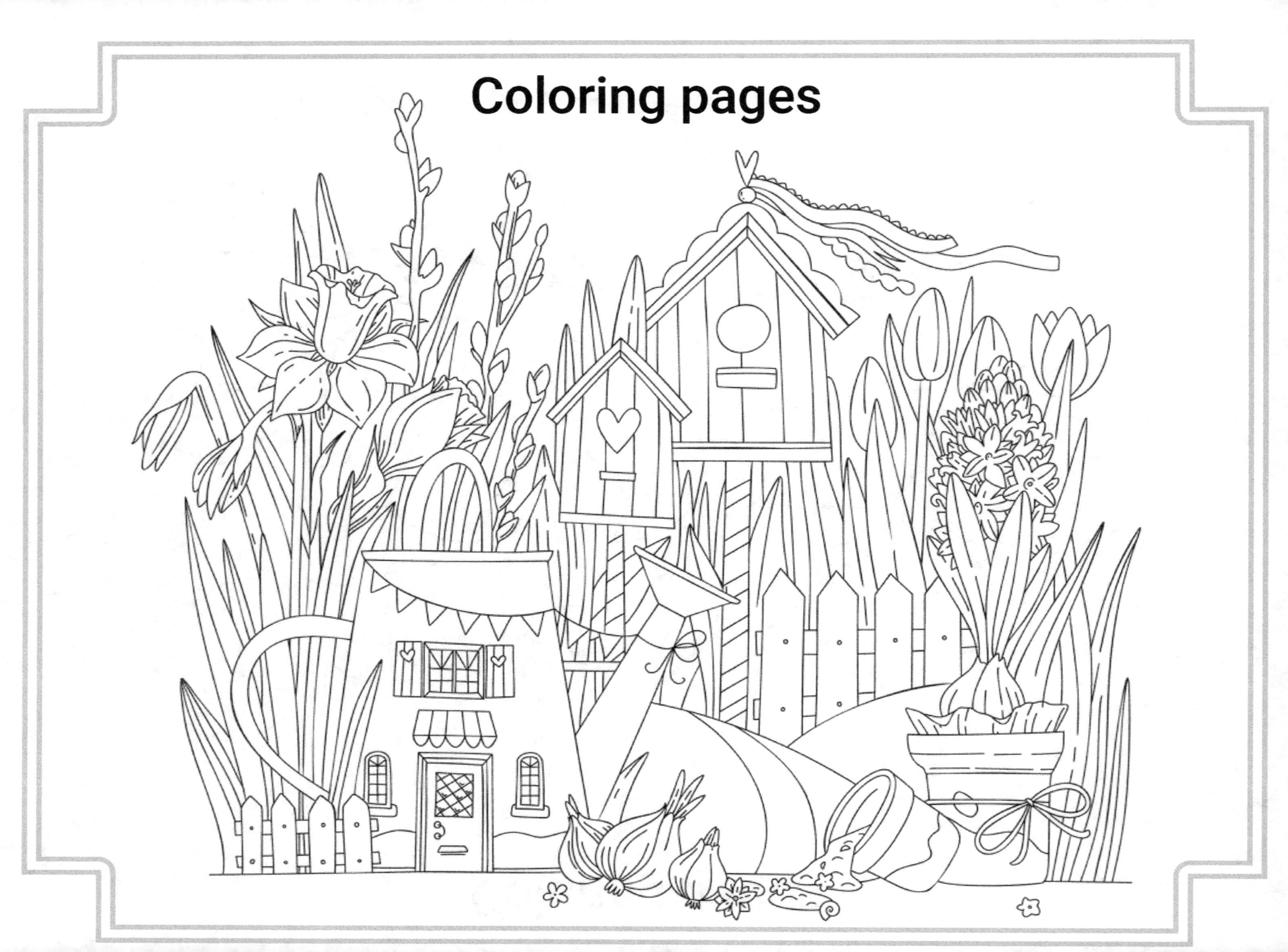

Coloring pages

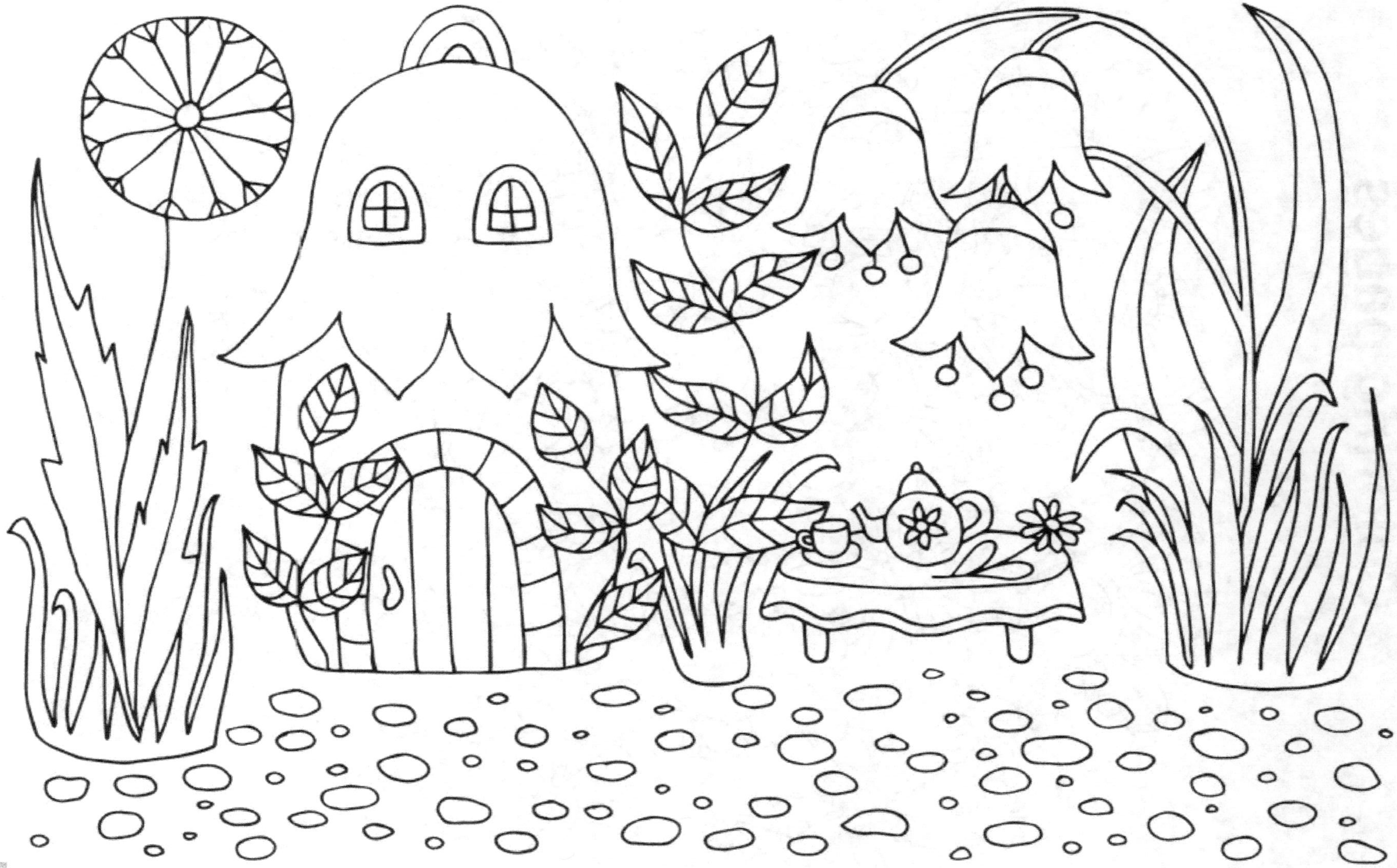

Coloring pages

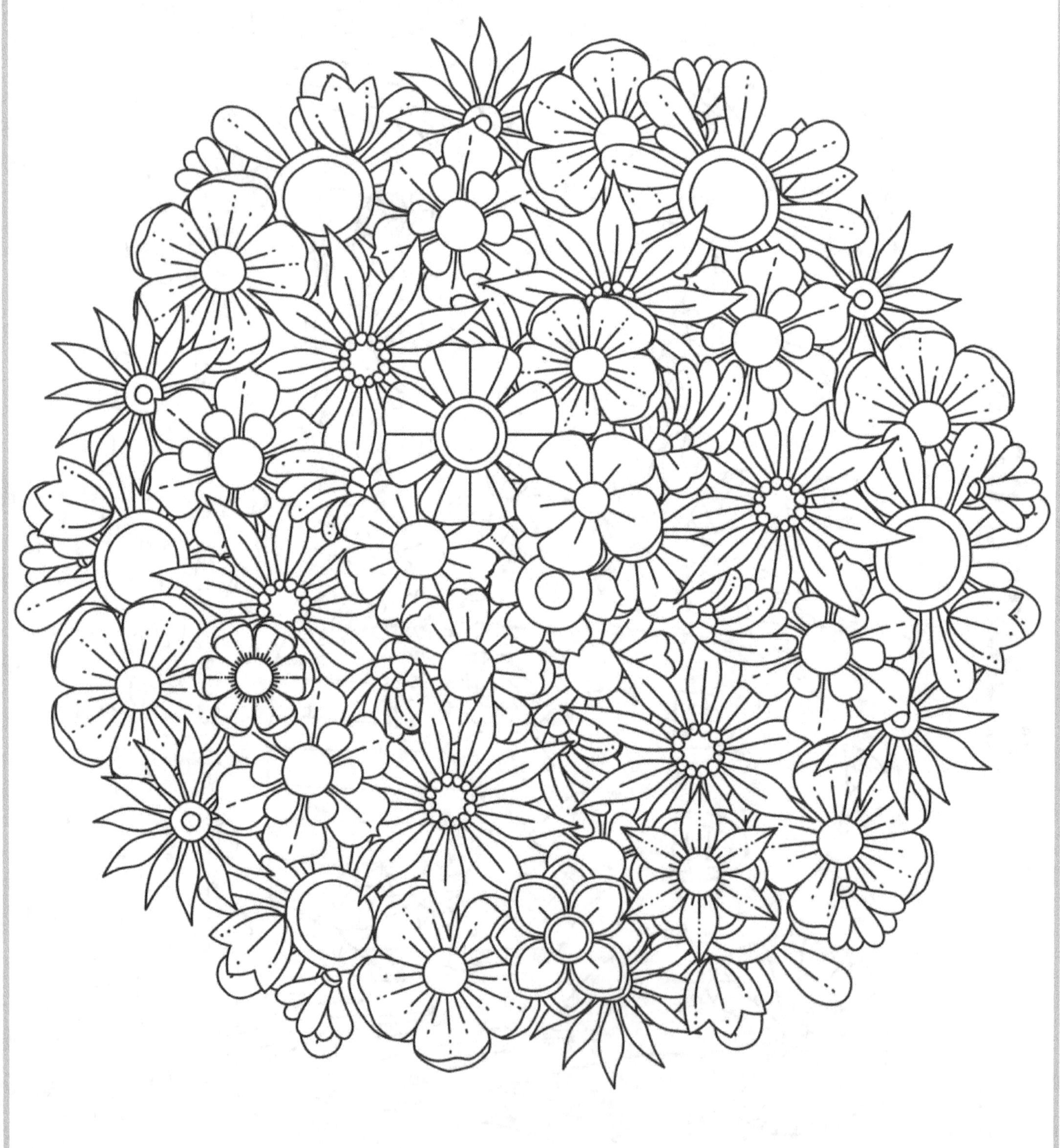

Coloring pages

Coloring pages

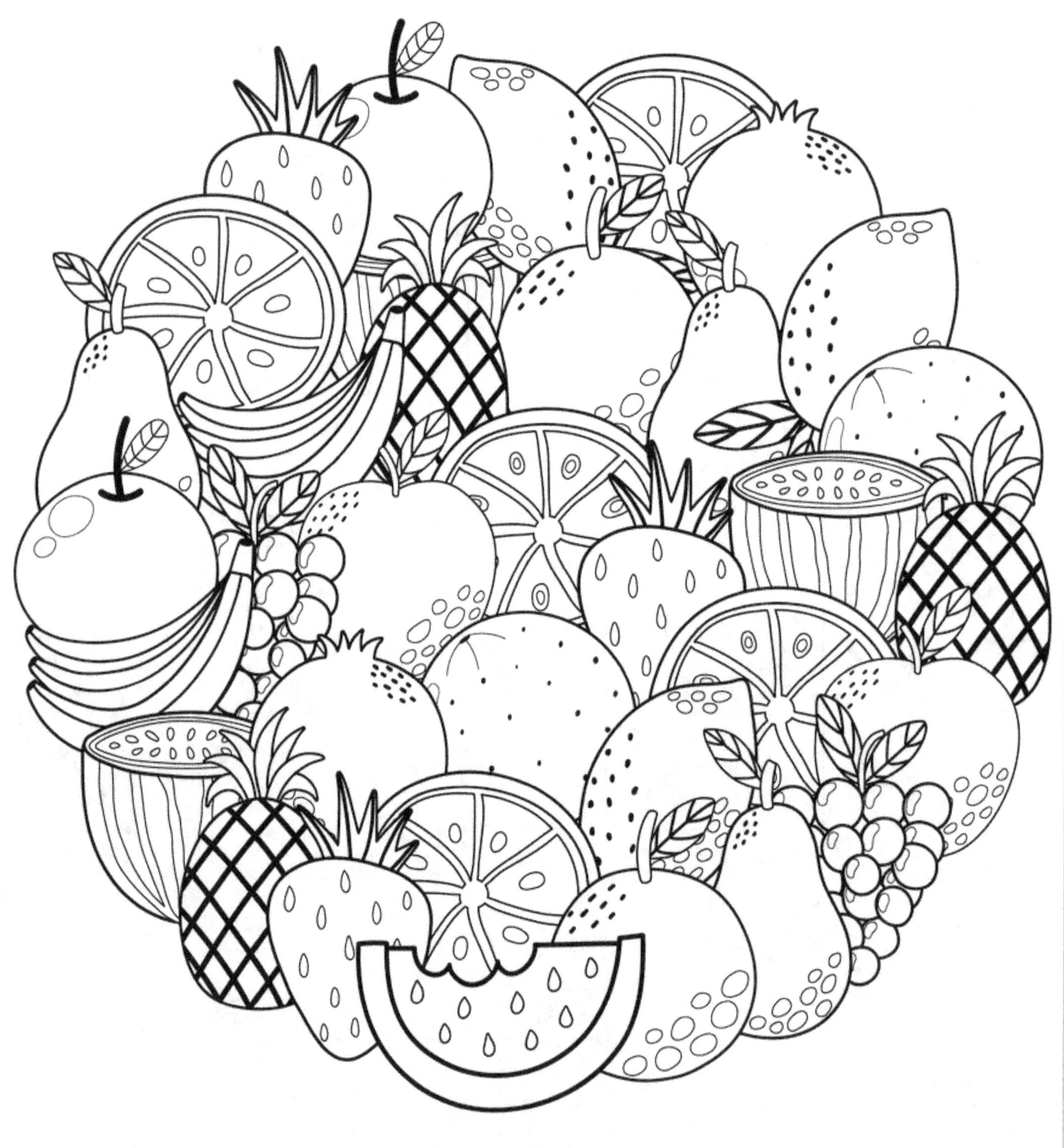

Coloring pages

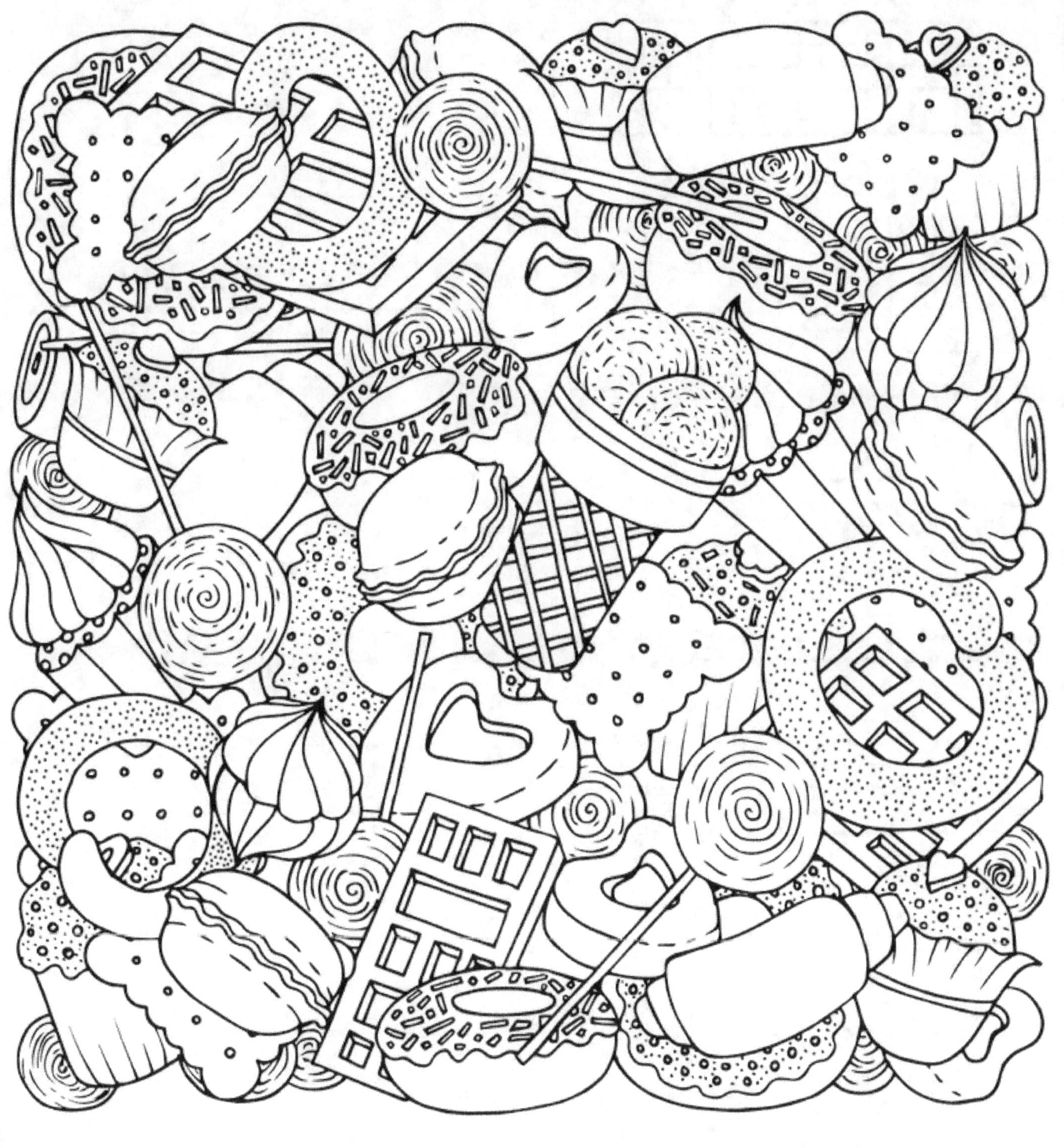

Continue the pattern

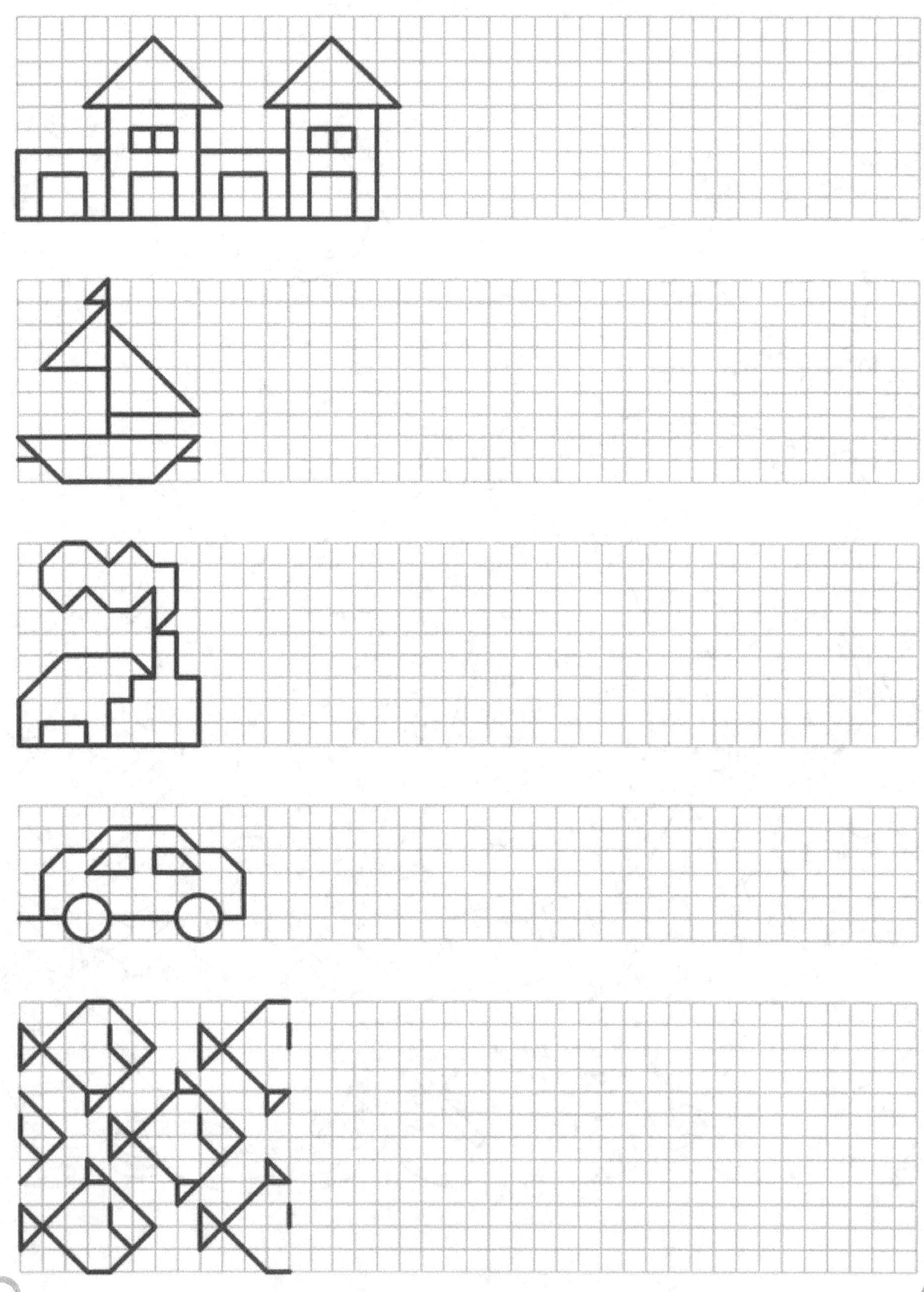

Continue the pattern

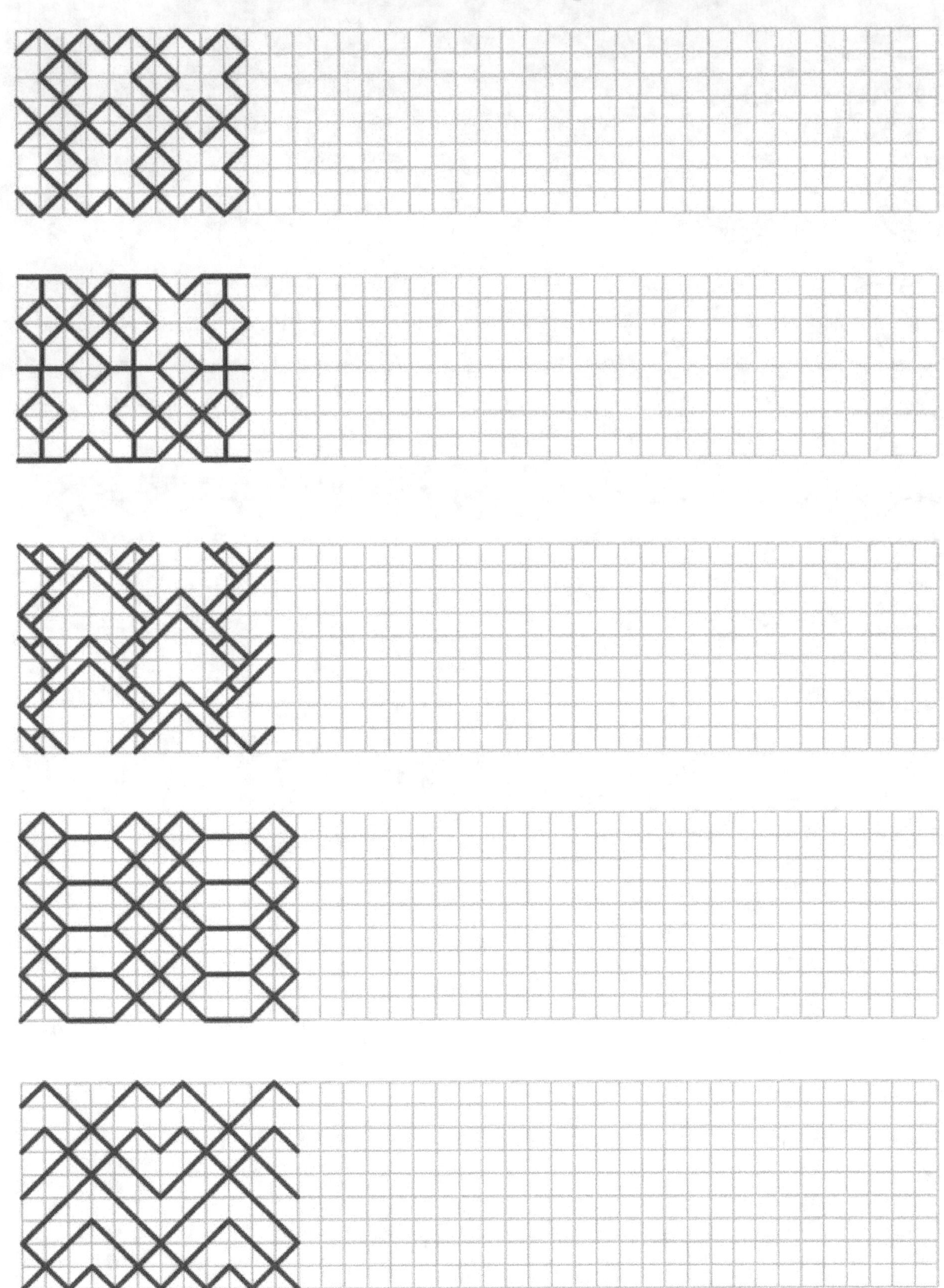

Continue the pattern

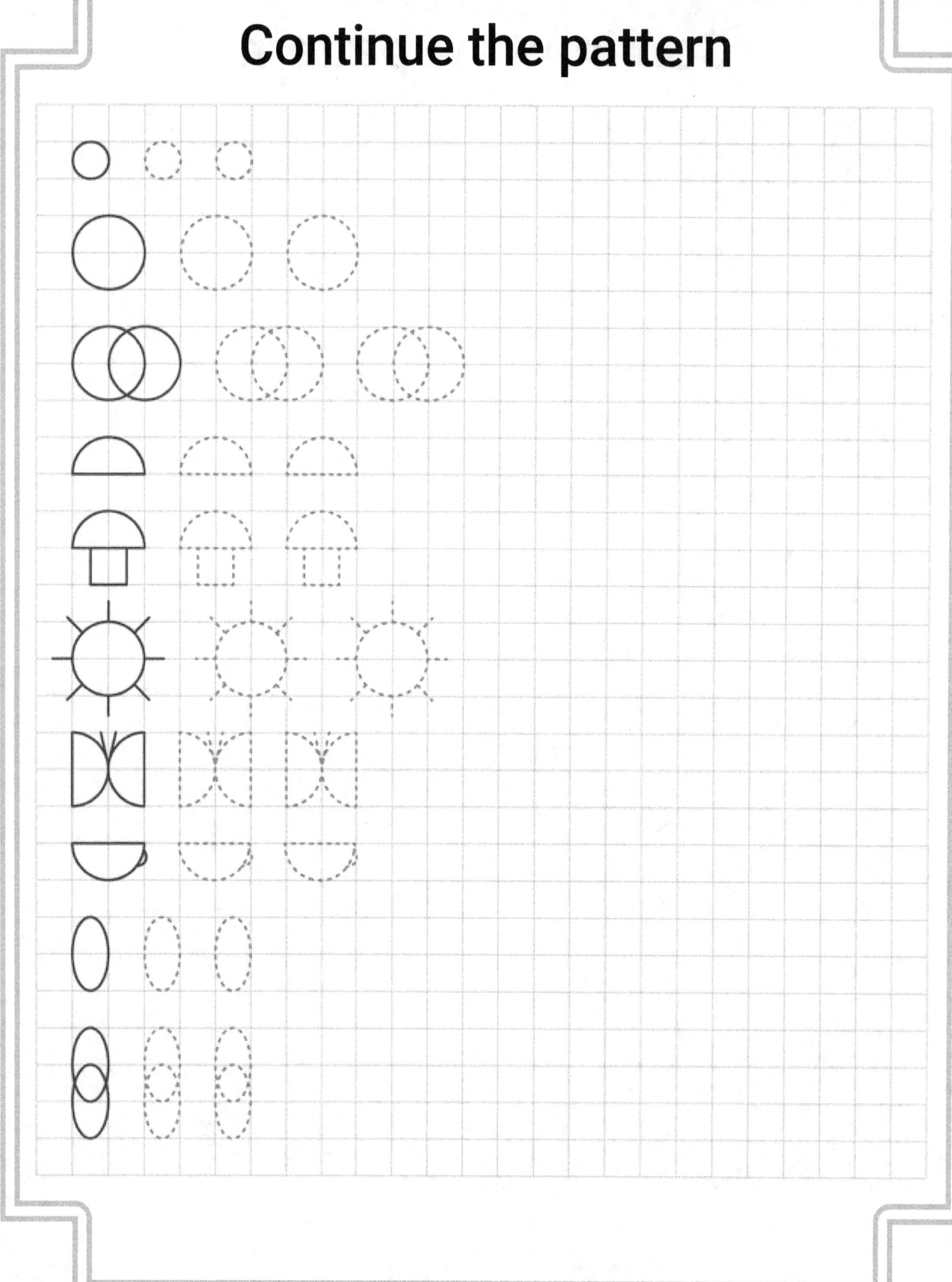

Eye-hand coordination

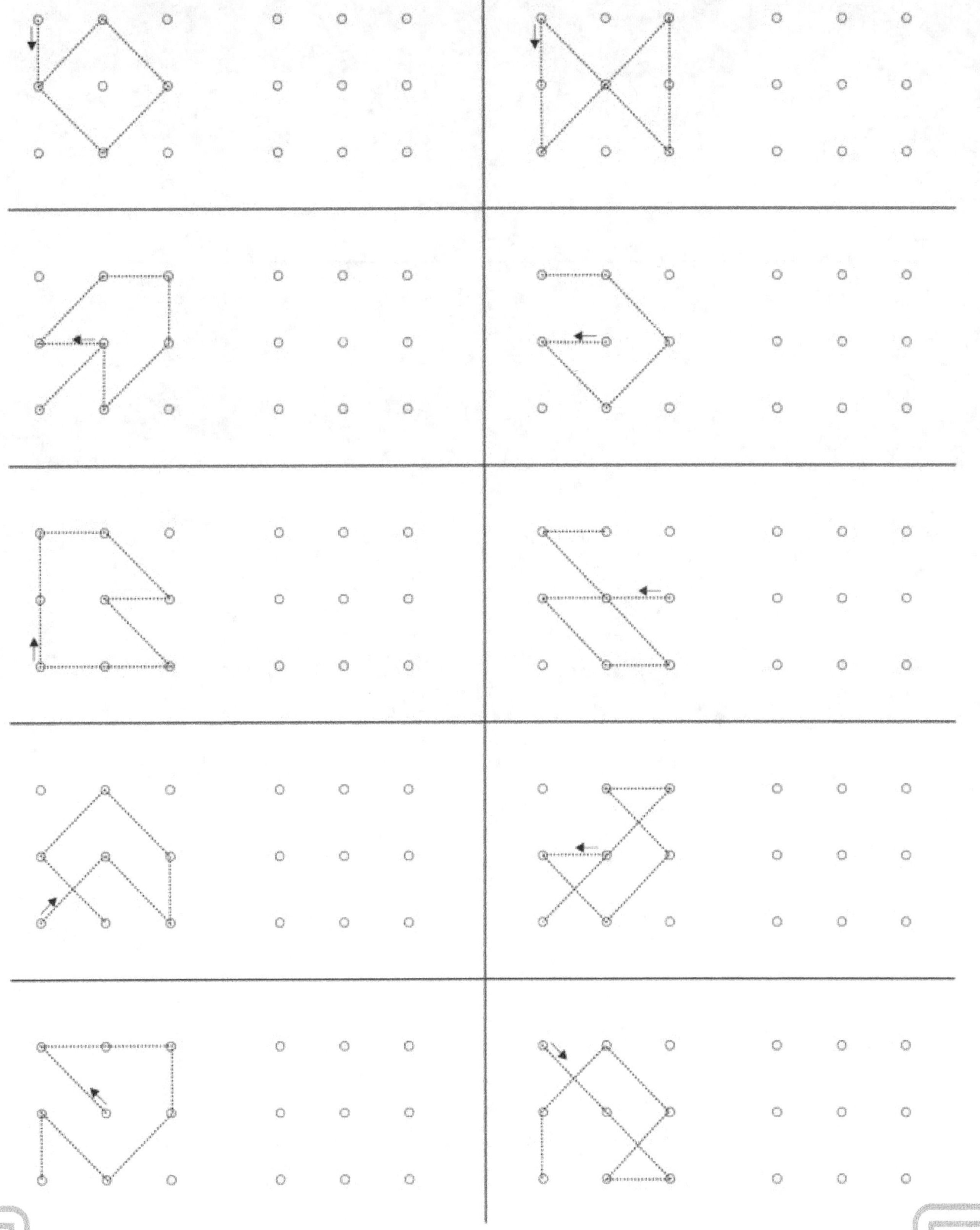

Eye-hand coordination

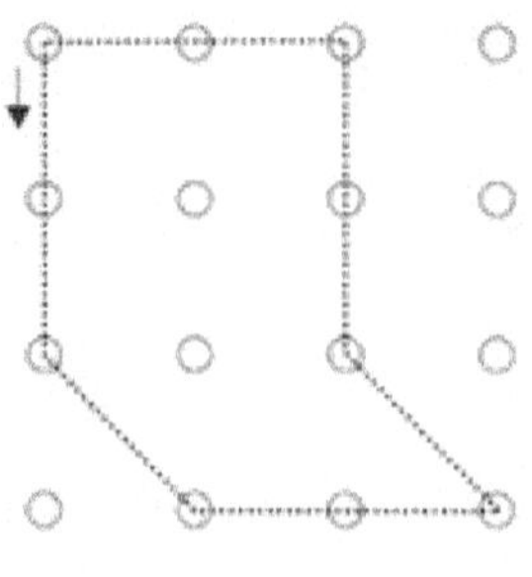 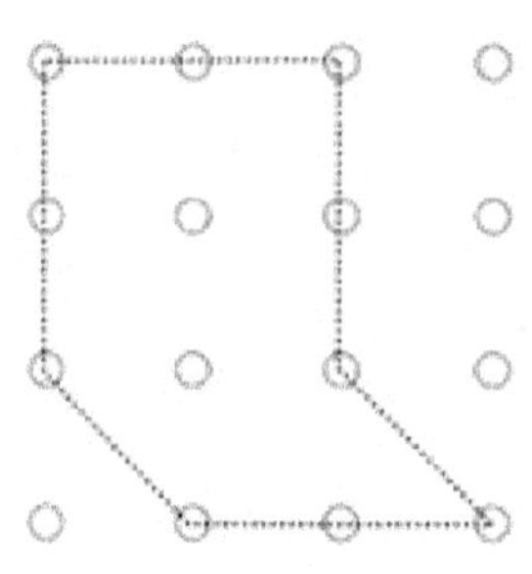 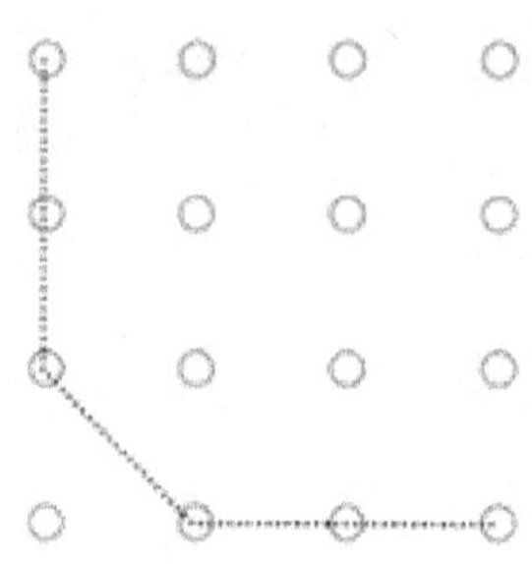

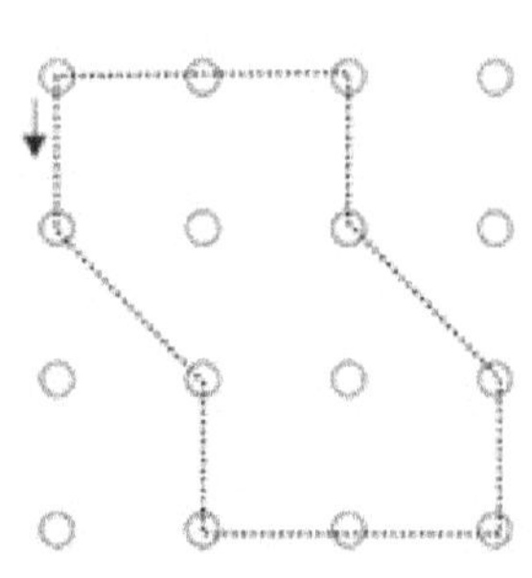 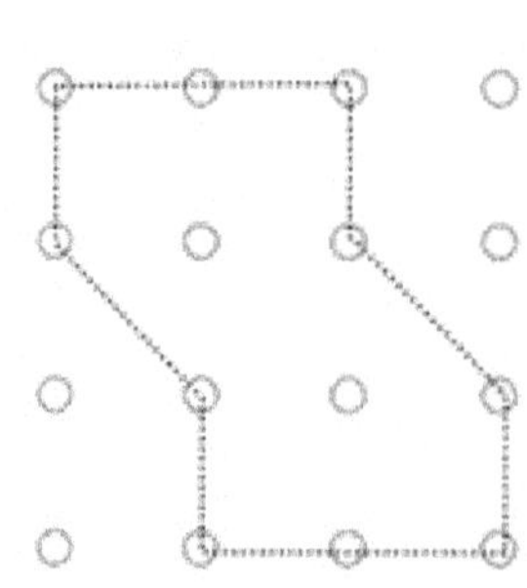 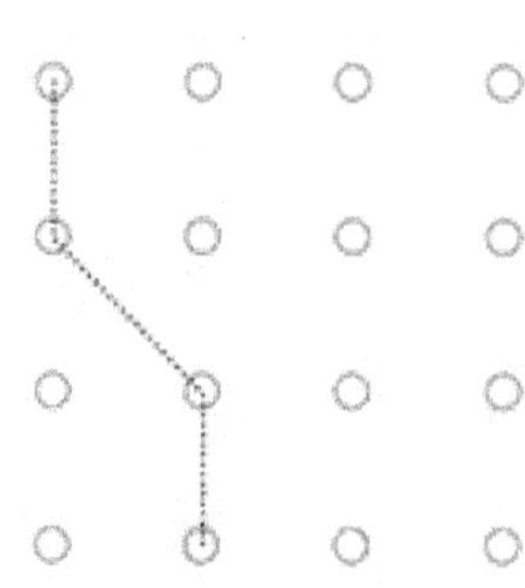

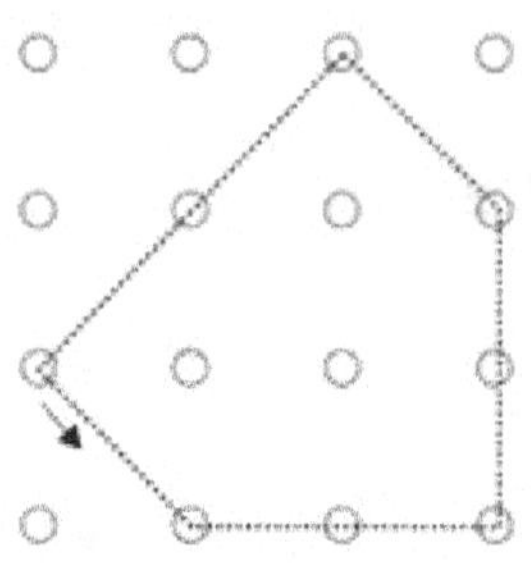 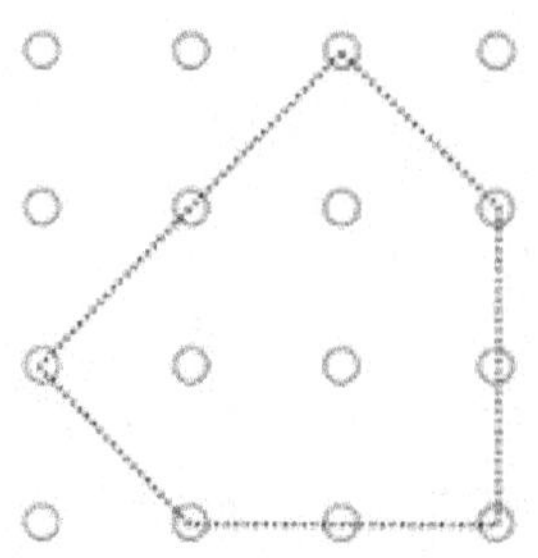 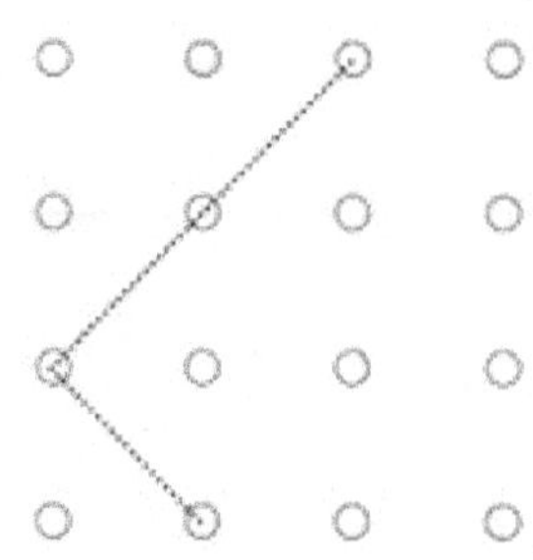

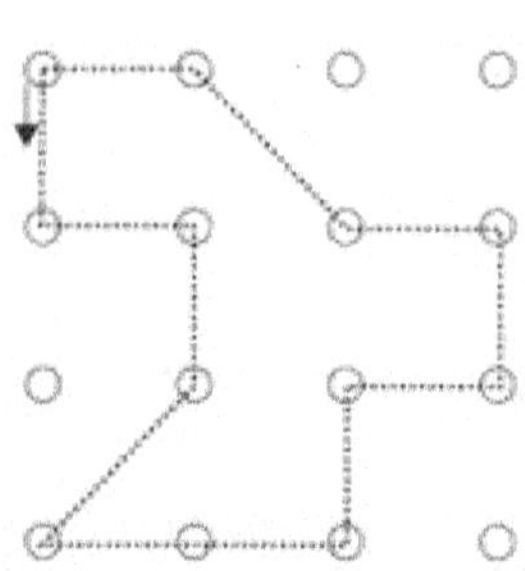 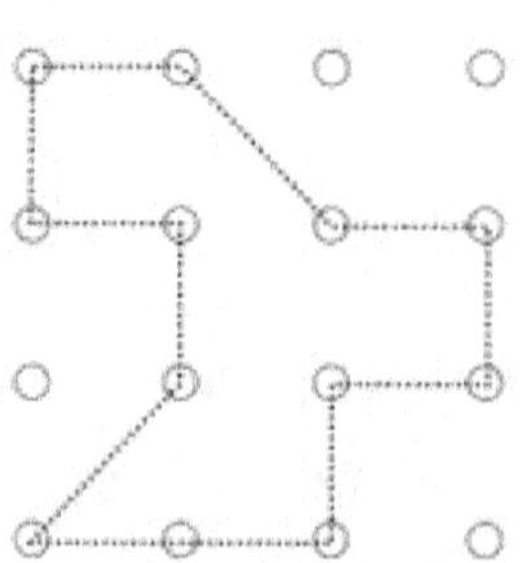 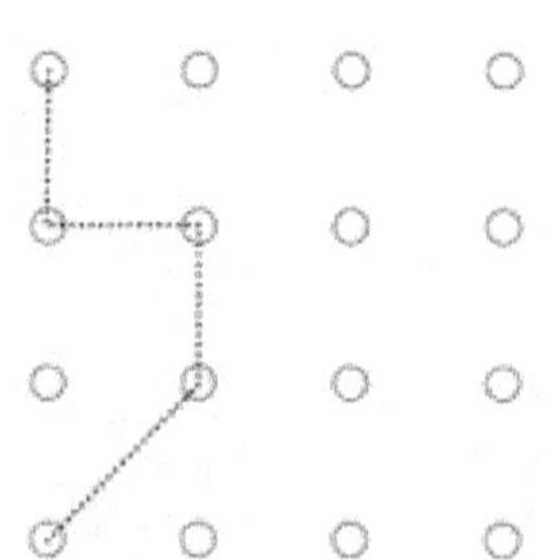

Eye-hand coordination

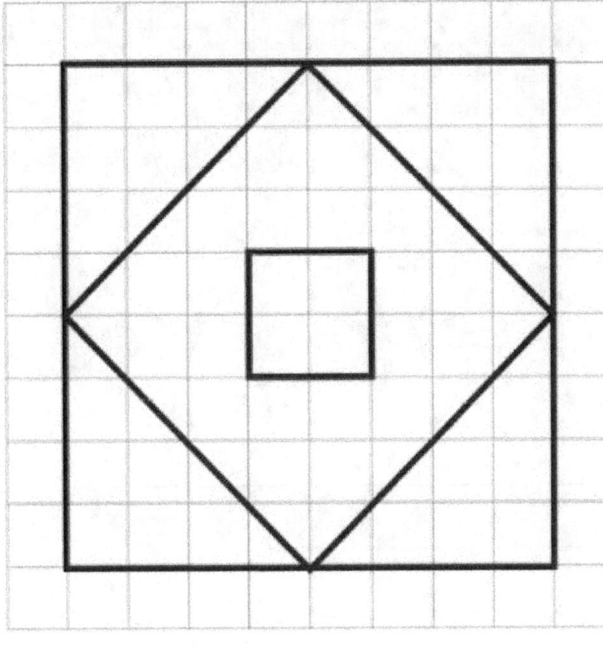

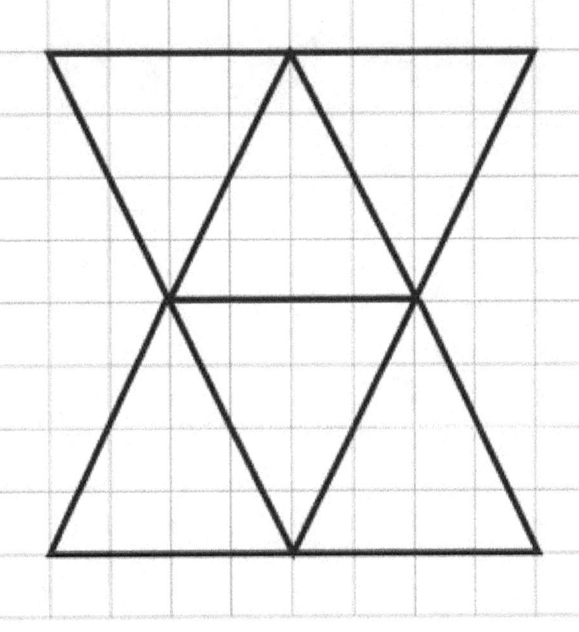

Eye-hand coordination

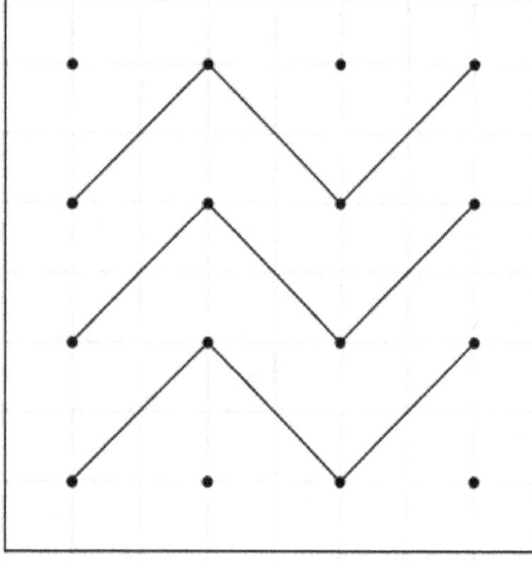
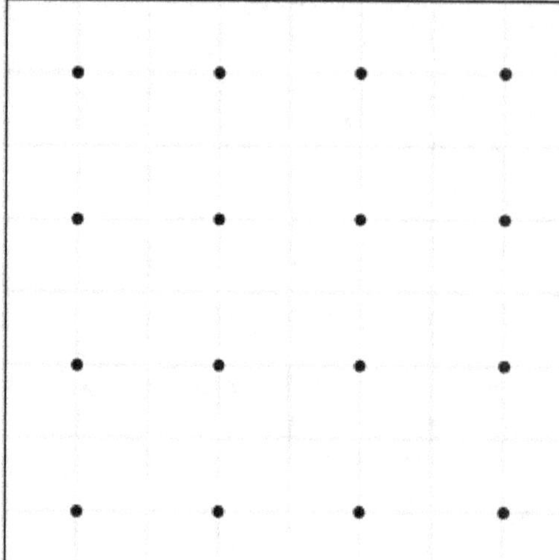
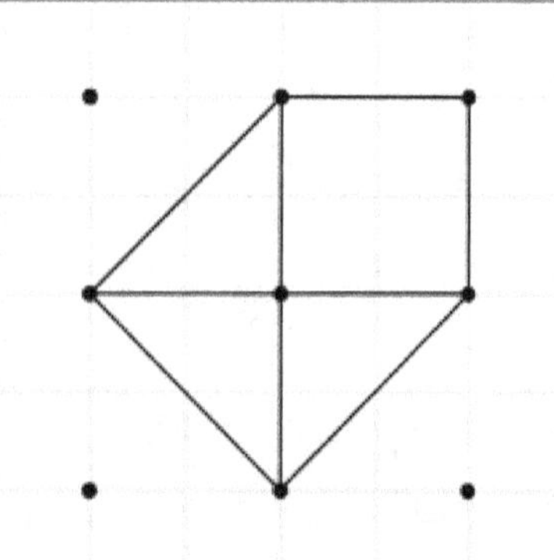
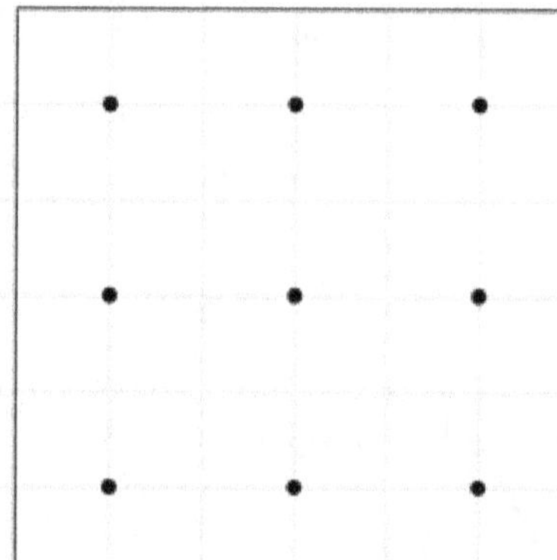
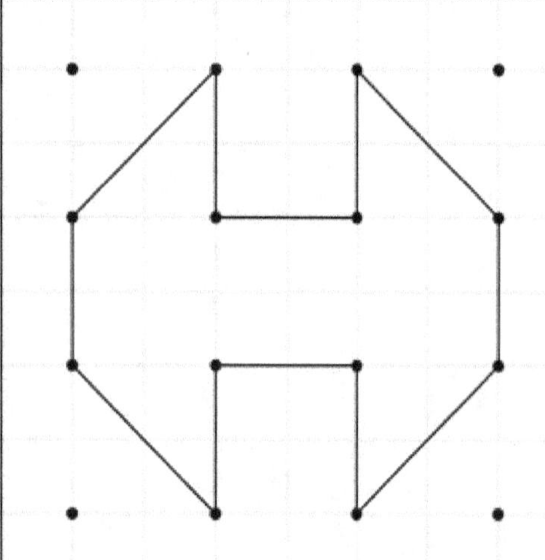
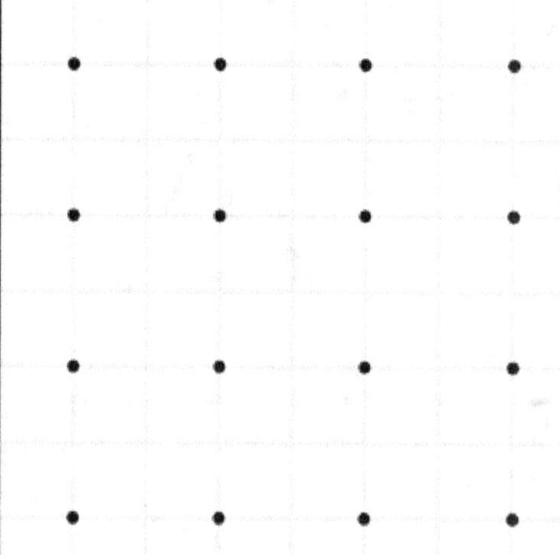

Eye-hand coordination

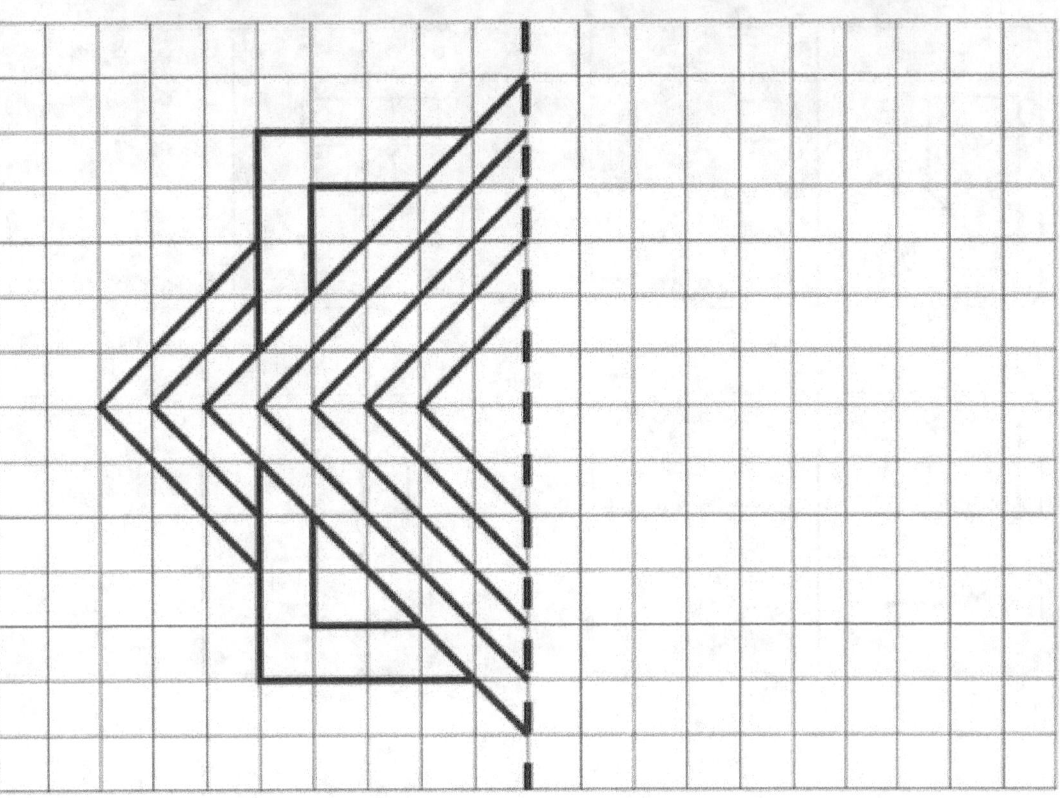

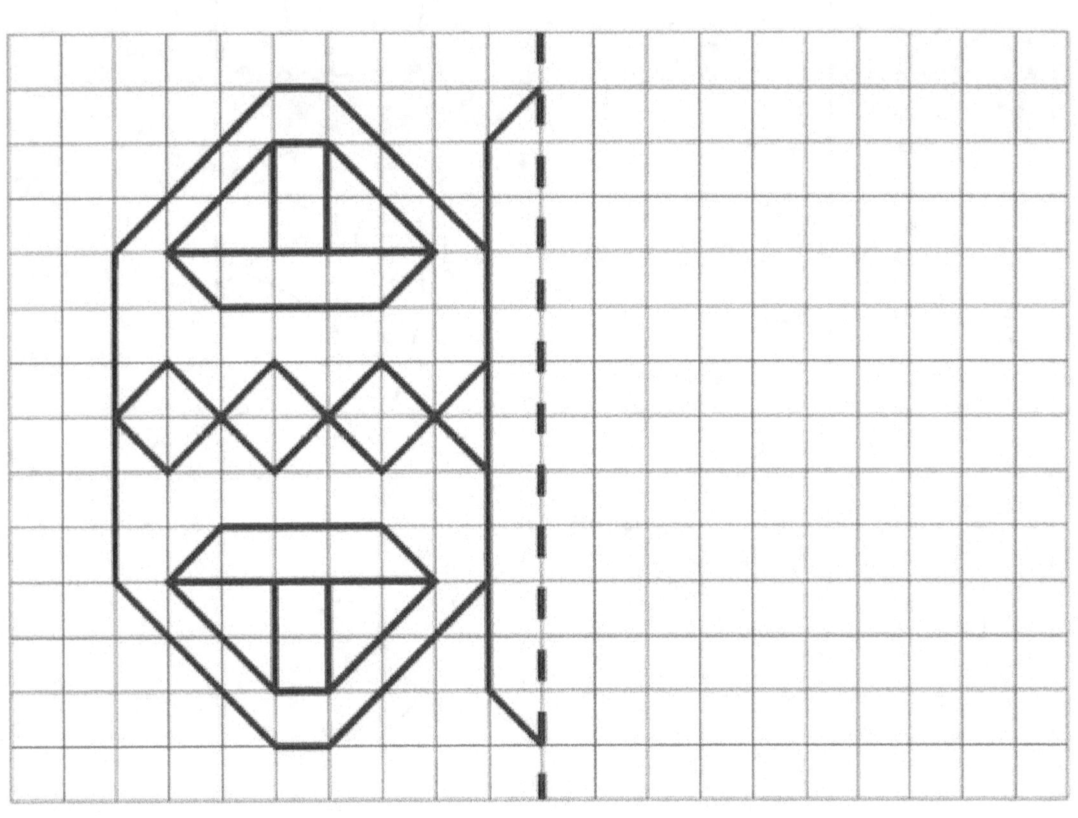

Eye-hand coordination

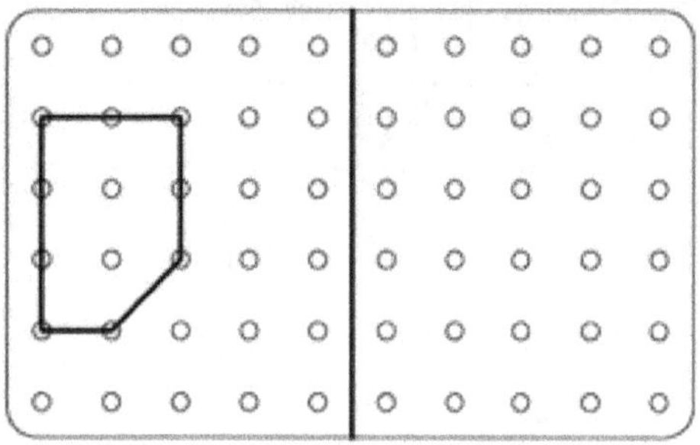 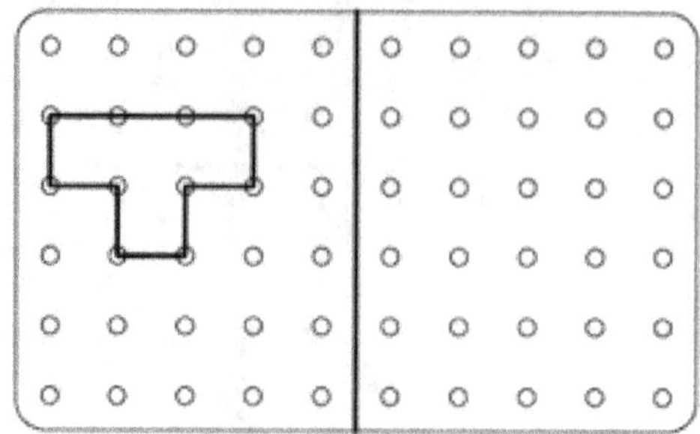

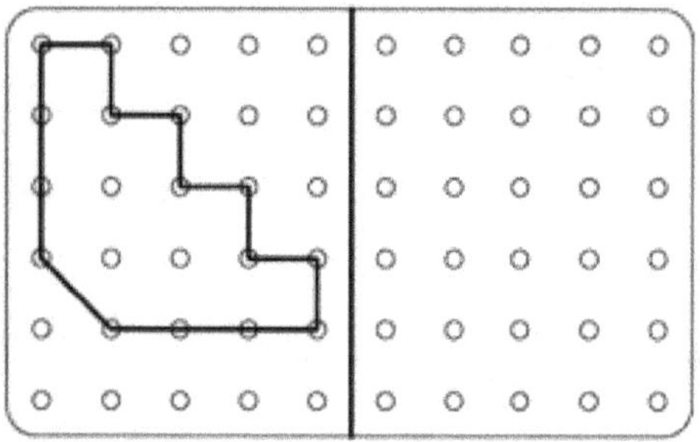 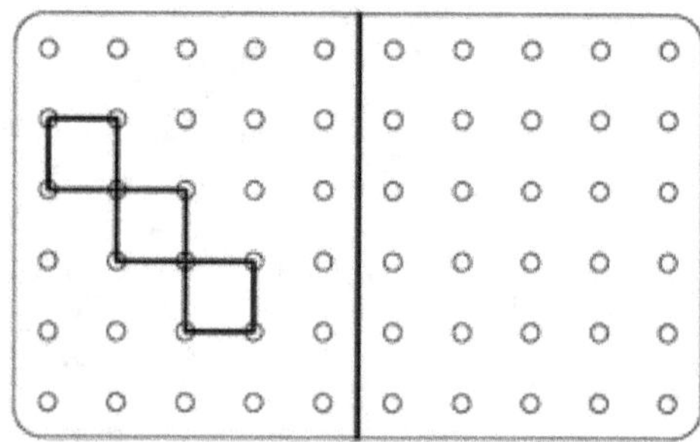

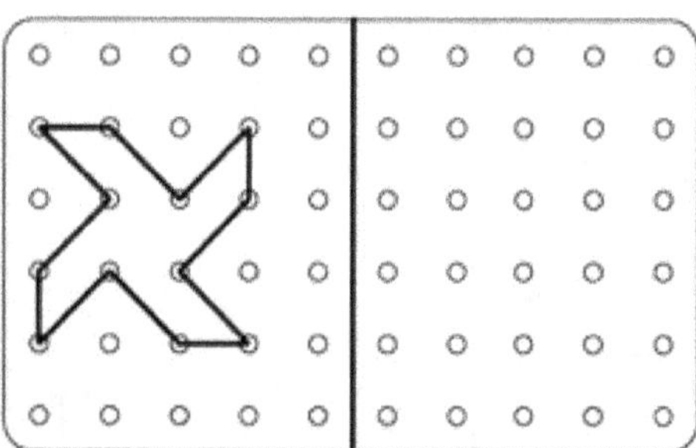 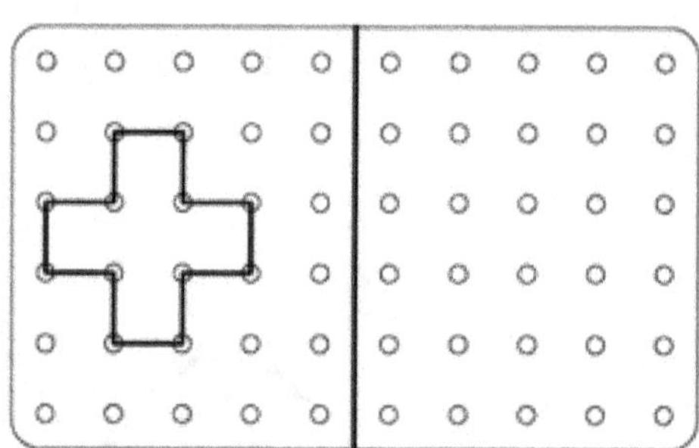

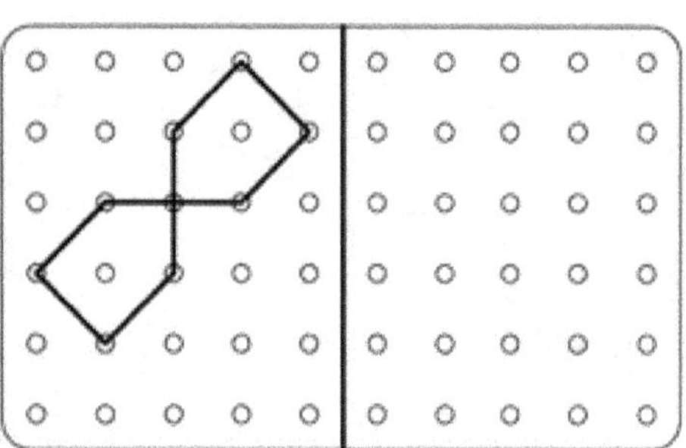 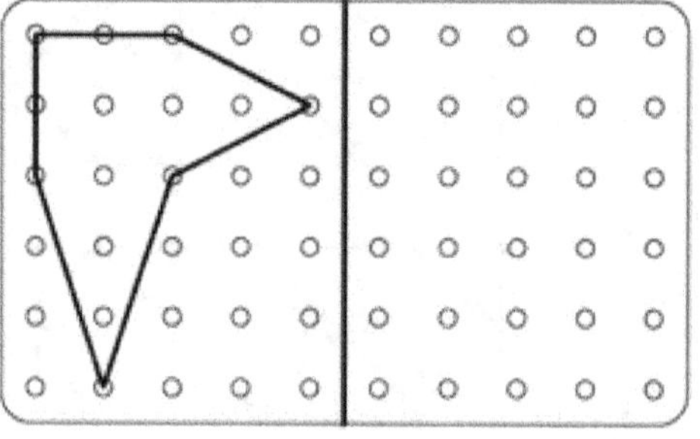

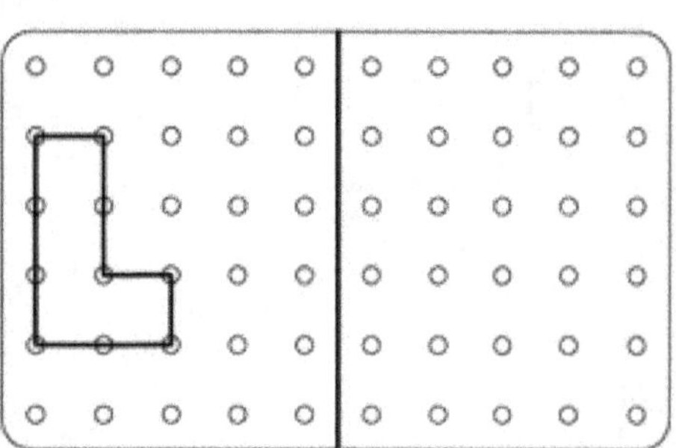 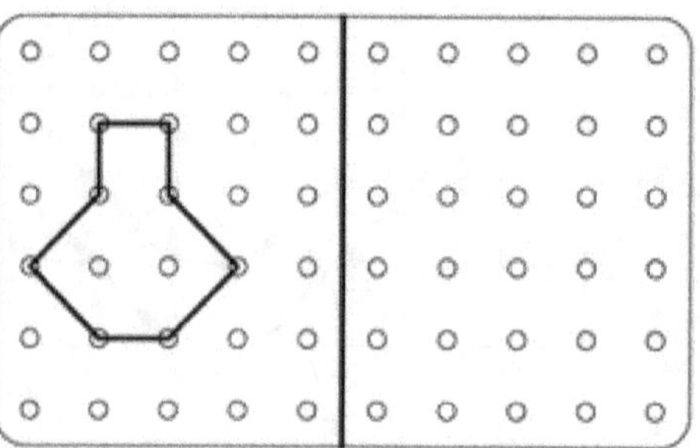

Find the ten differences between the two pictures.

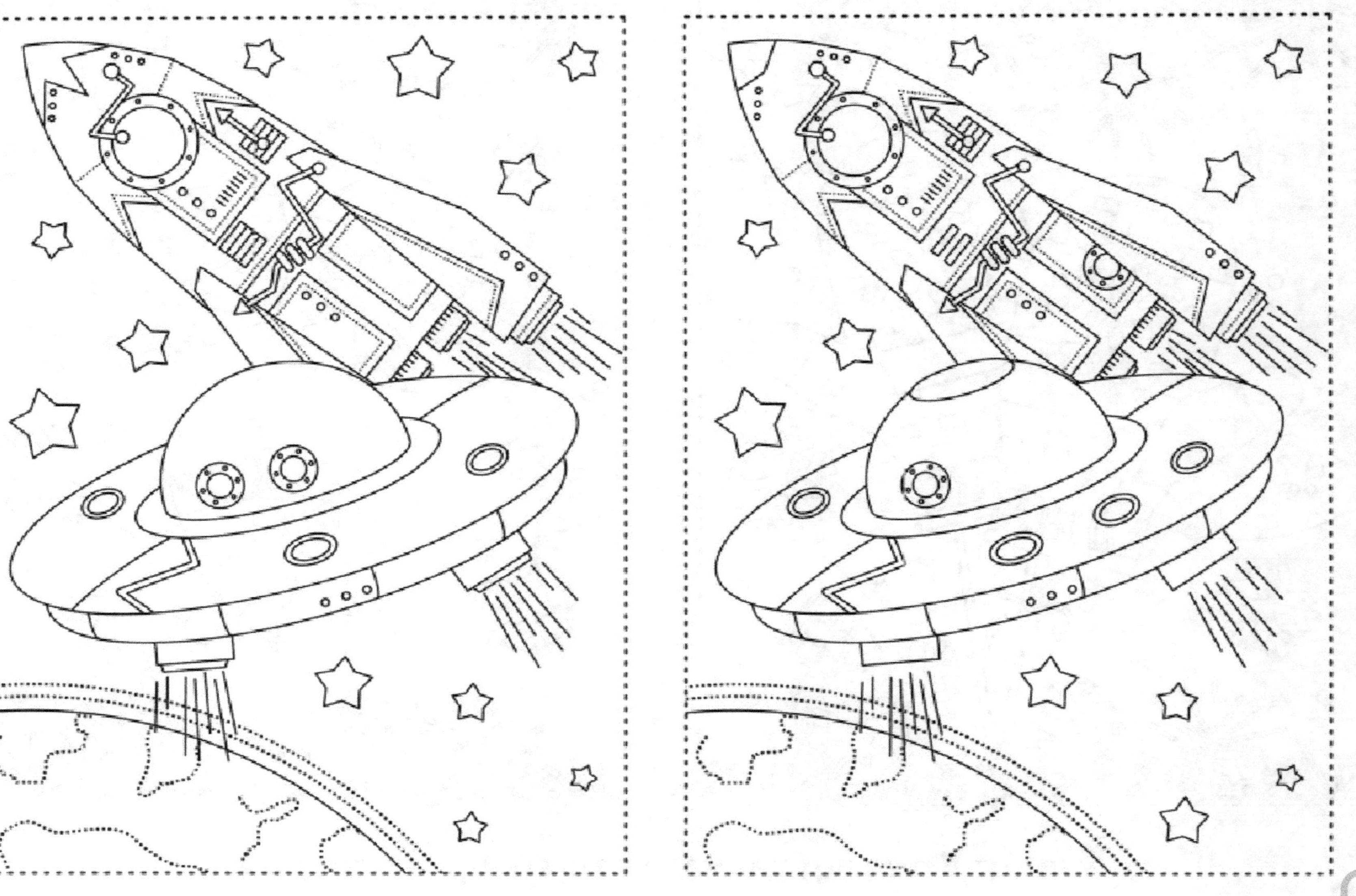

Find the ten differences between the two pictures.

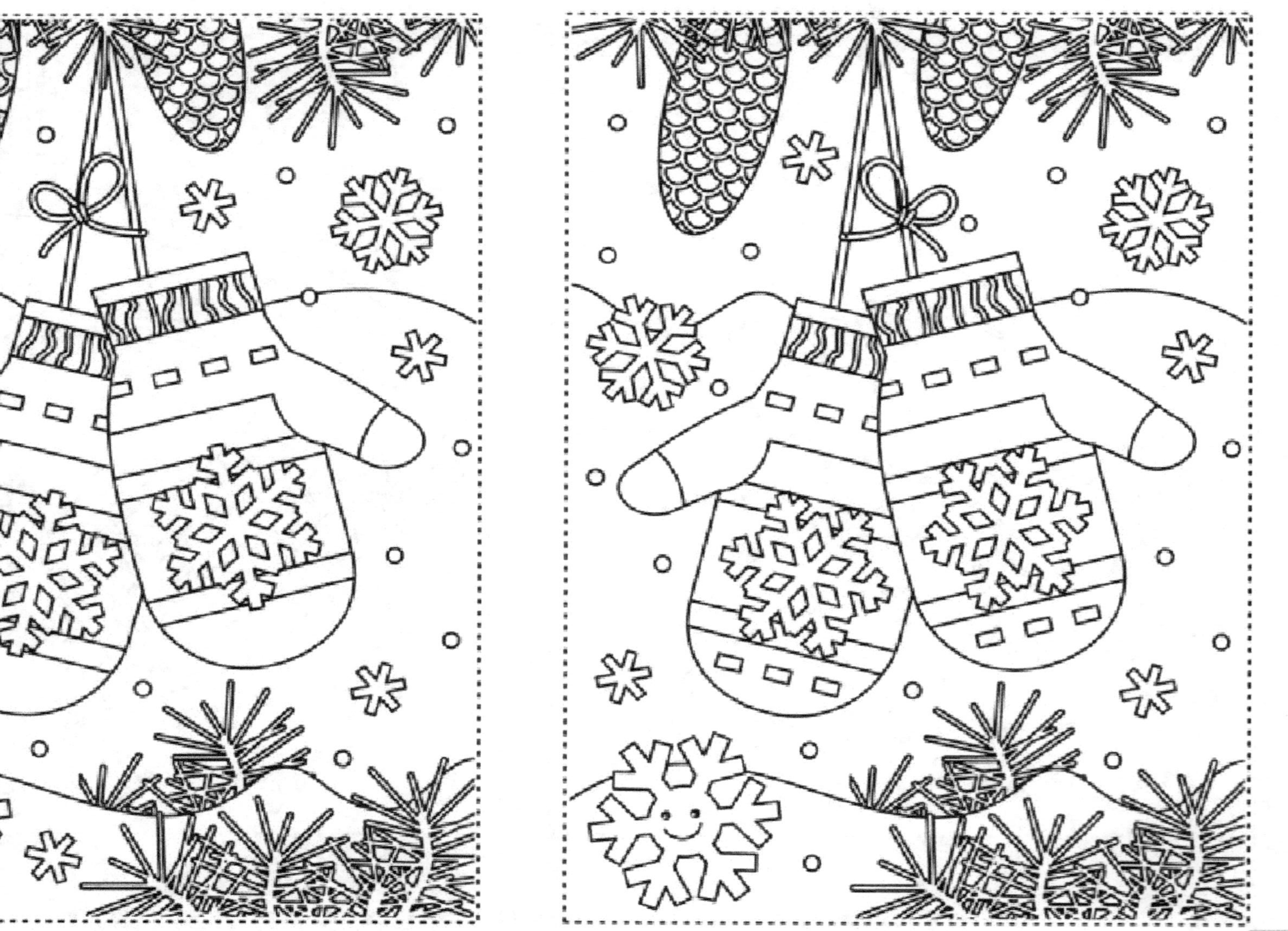

Find the ten differences between the two pictures.

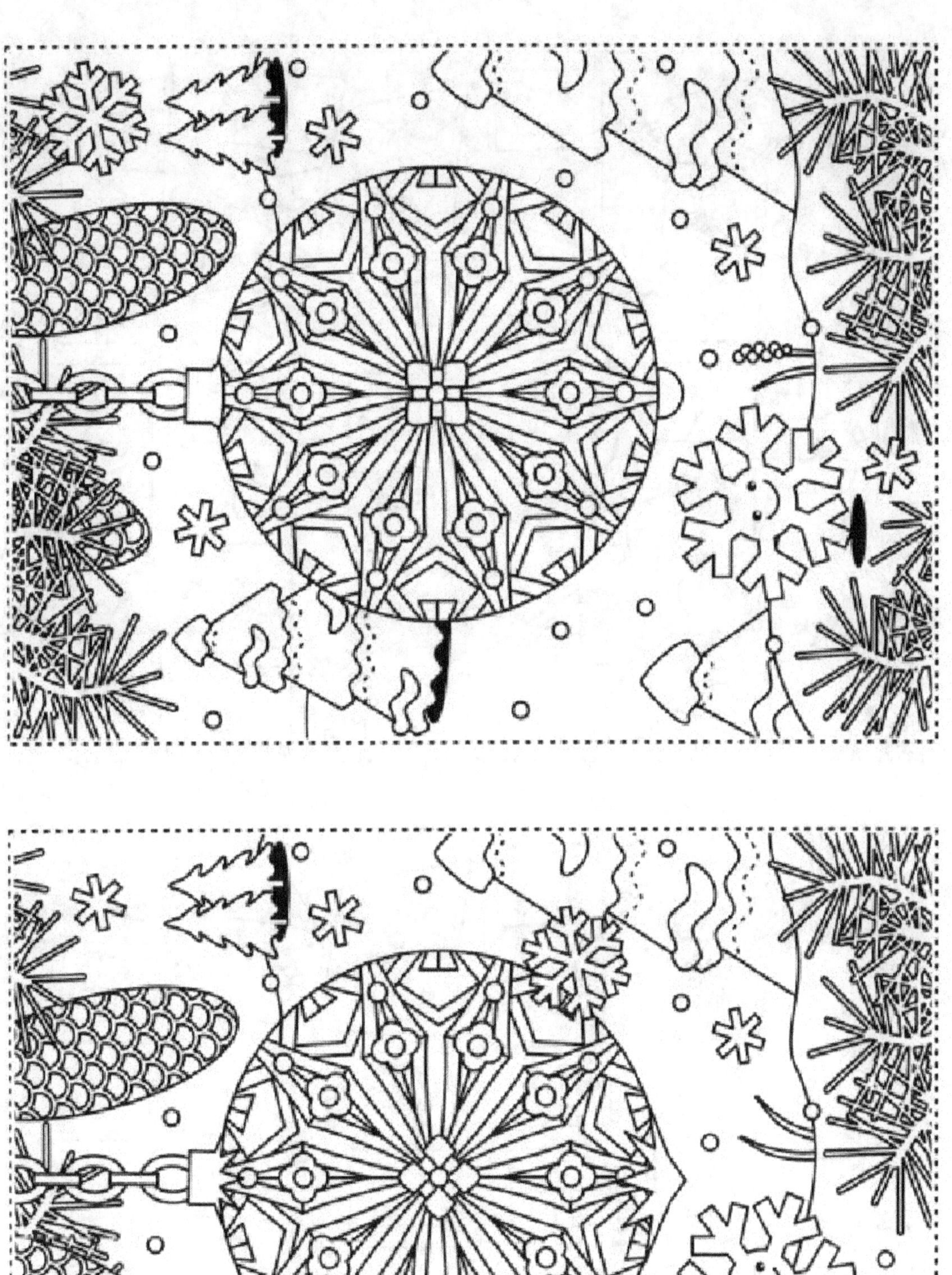

Find 10 differences.

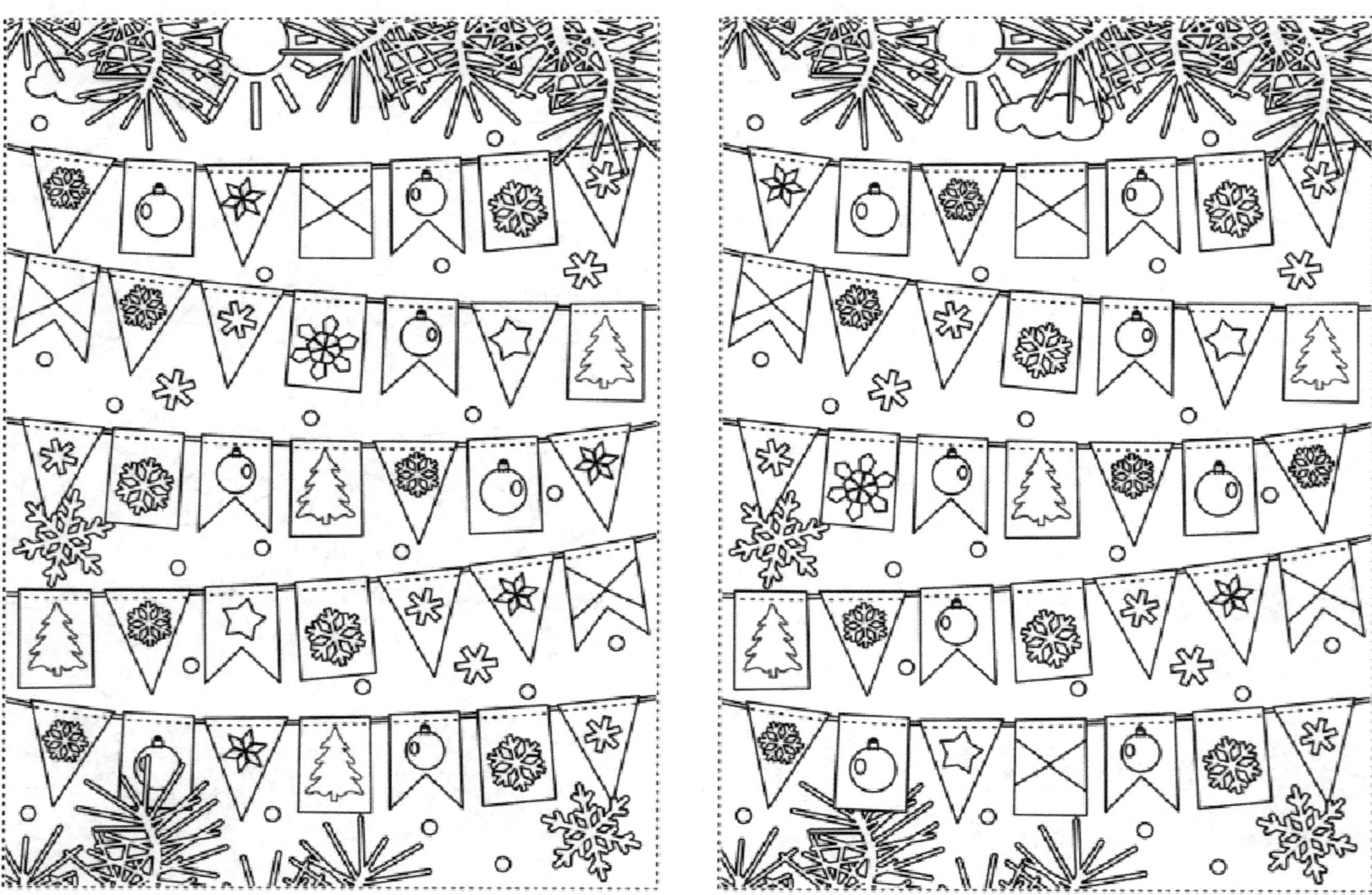

Find 10 differences.

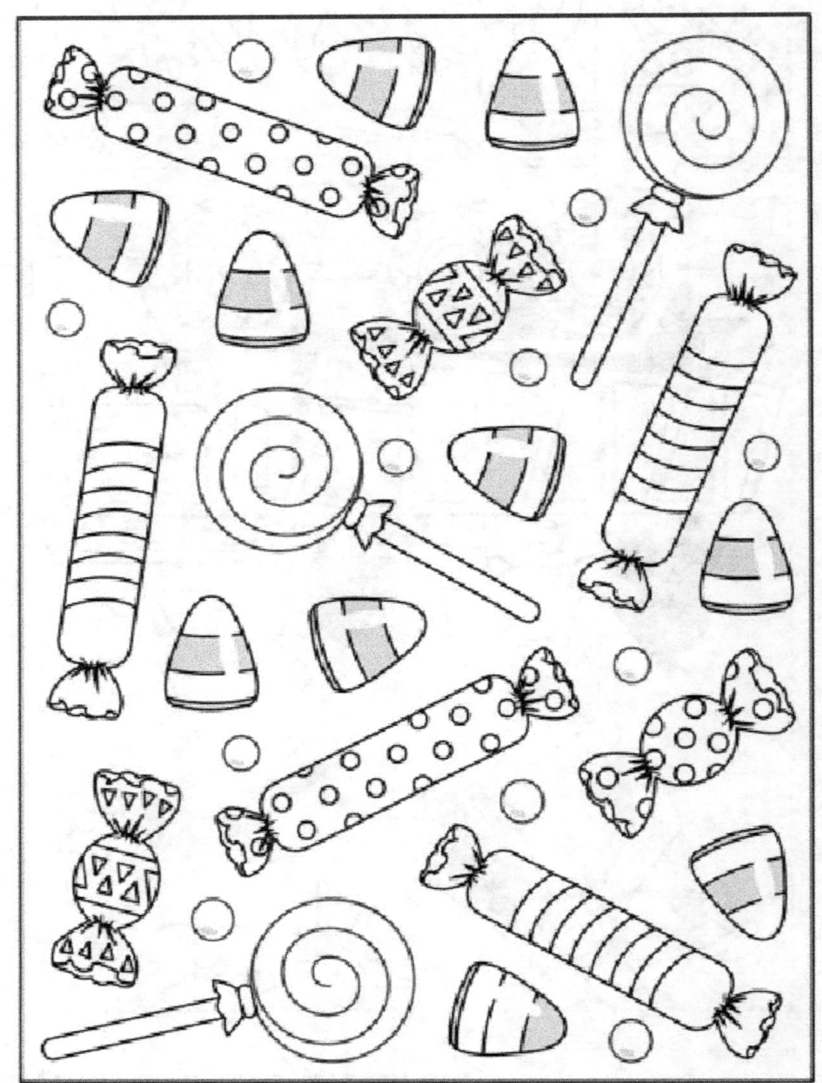

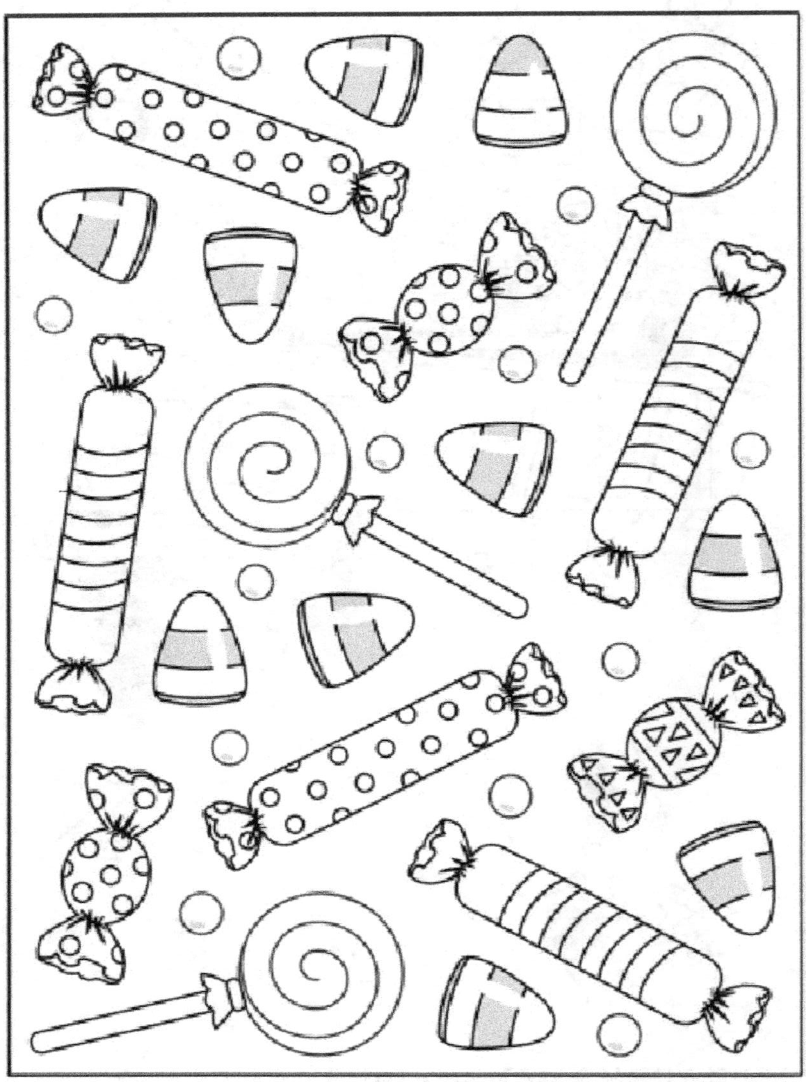

Find the ten differences between the two pictures.

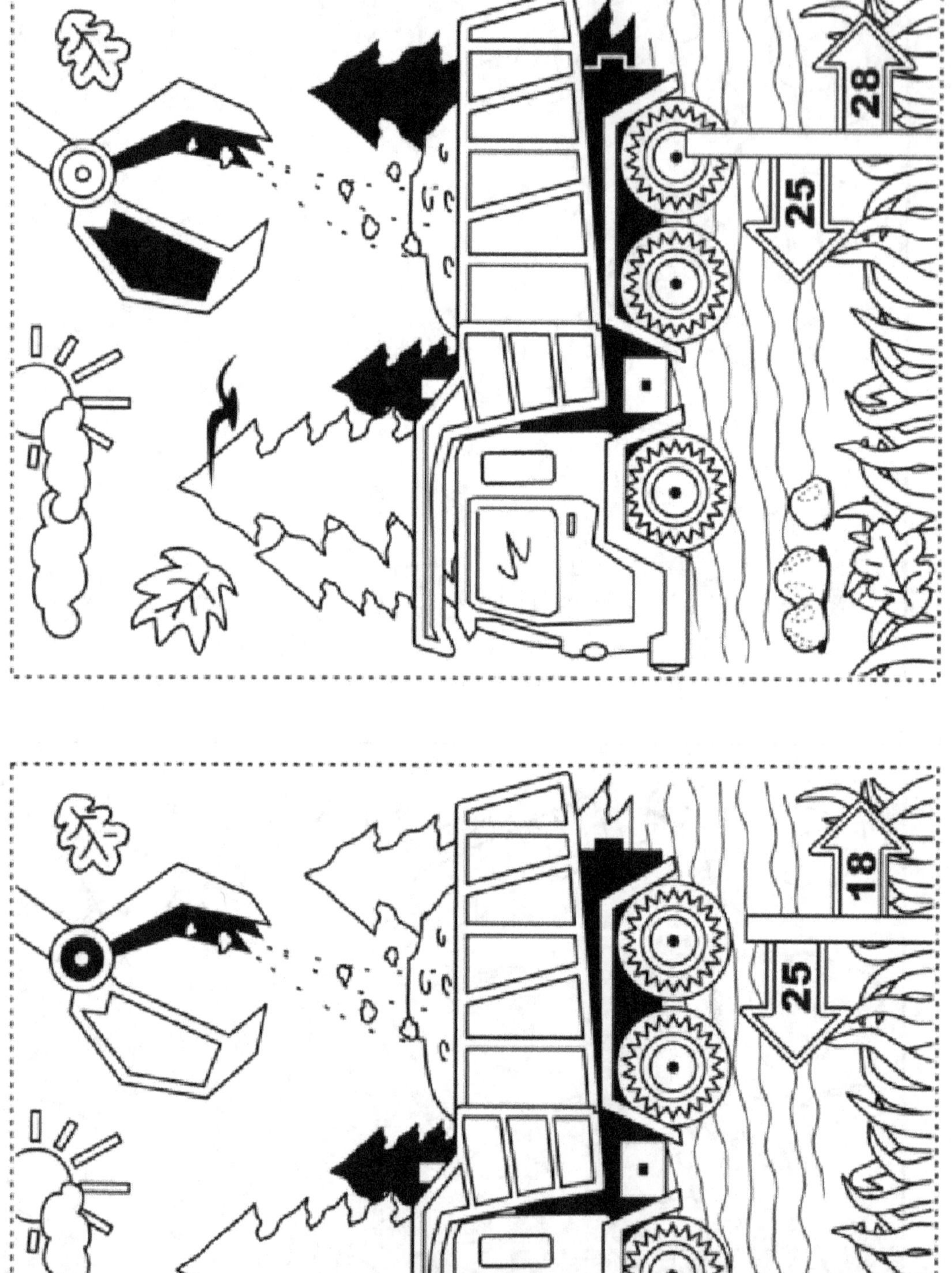

Find 5 differences

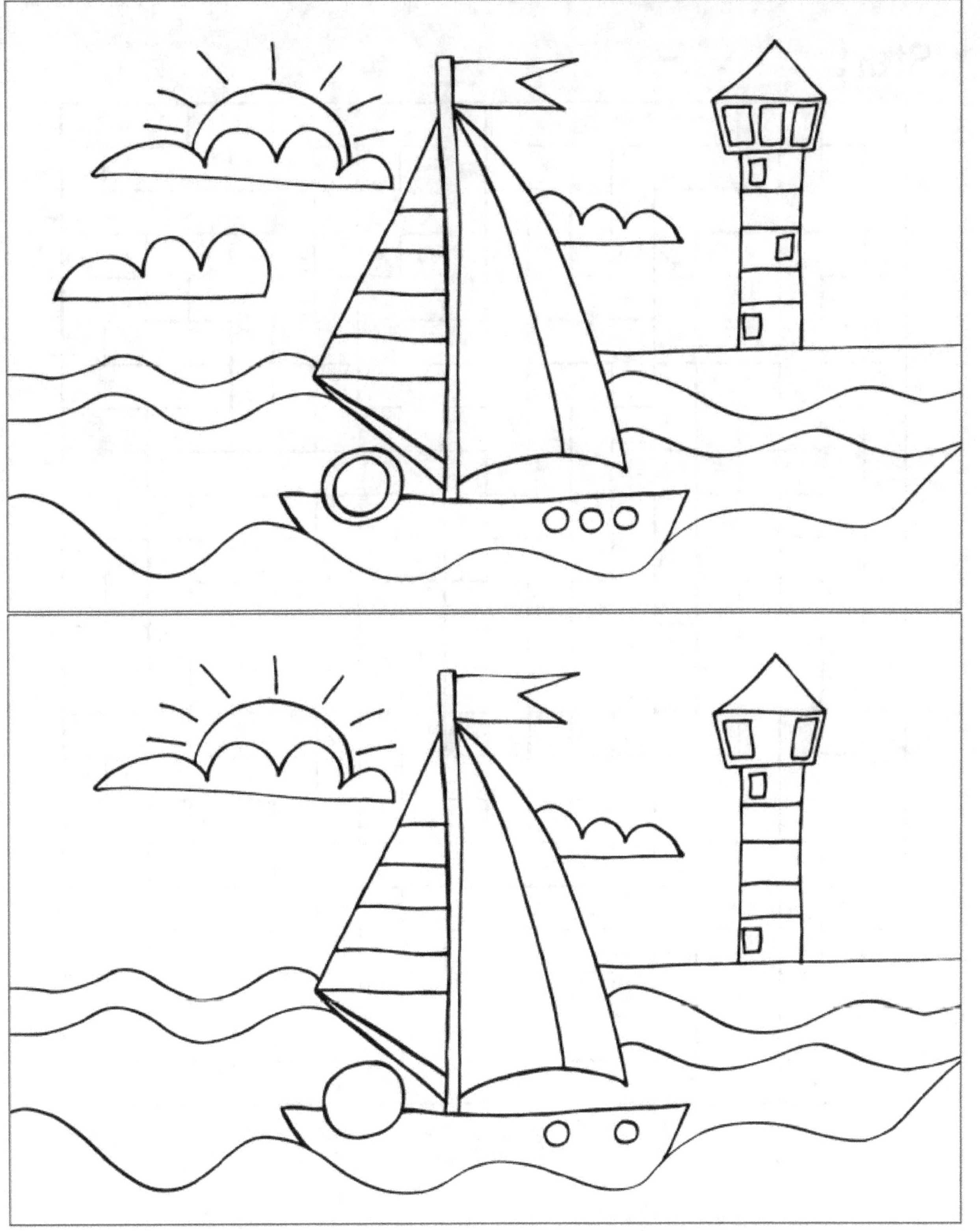

Maze 1

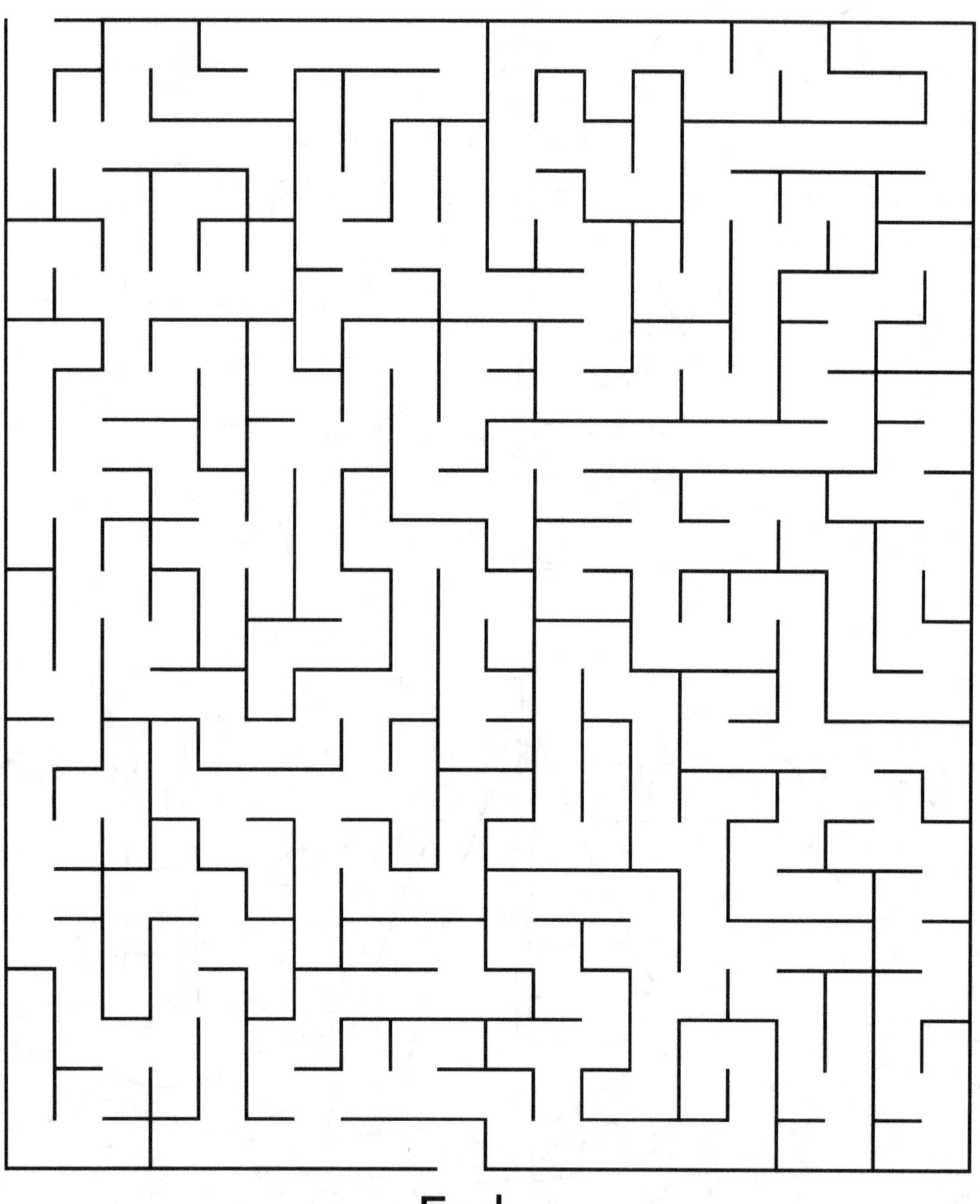

Maze 2

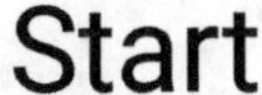

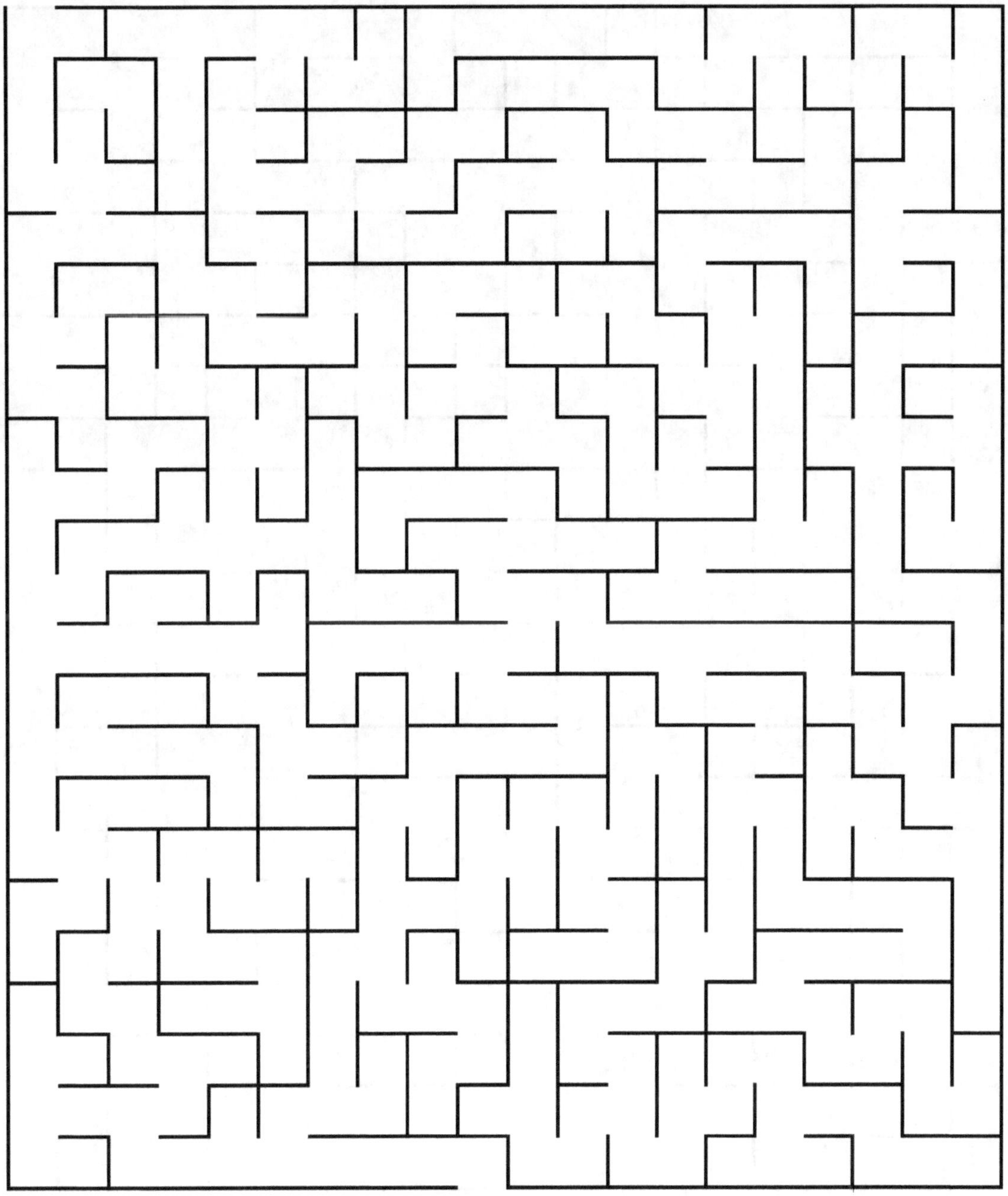

Maze 3

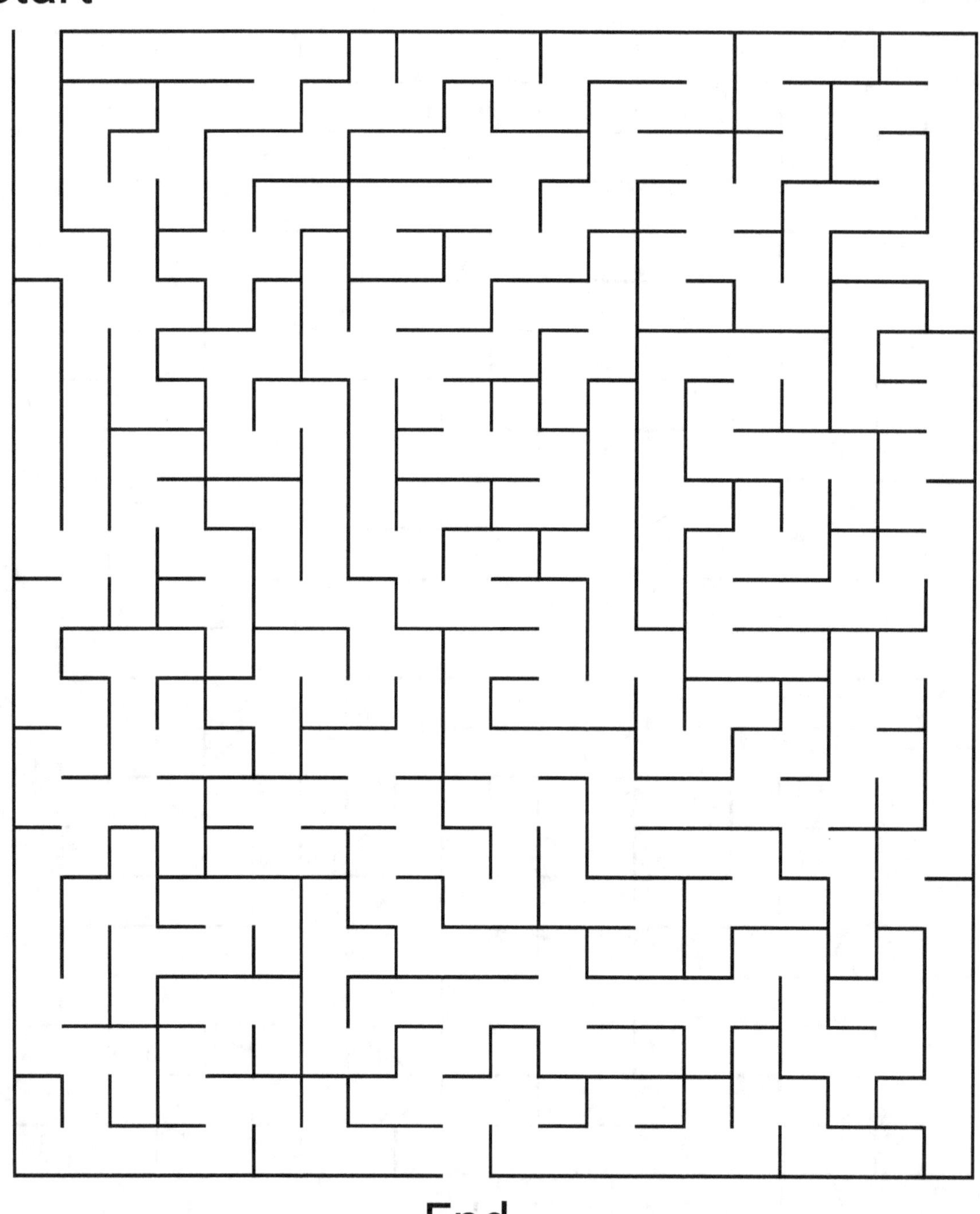

Maze 4

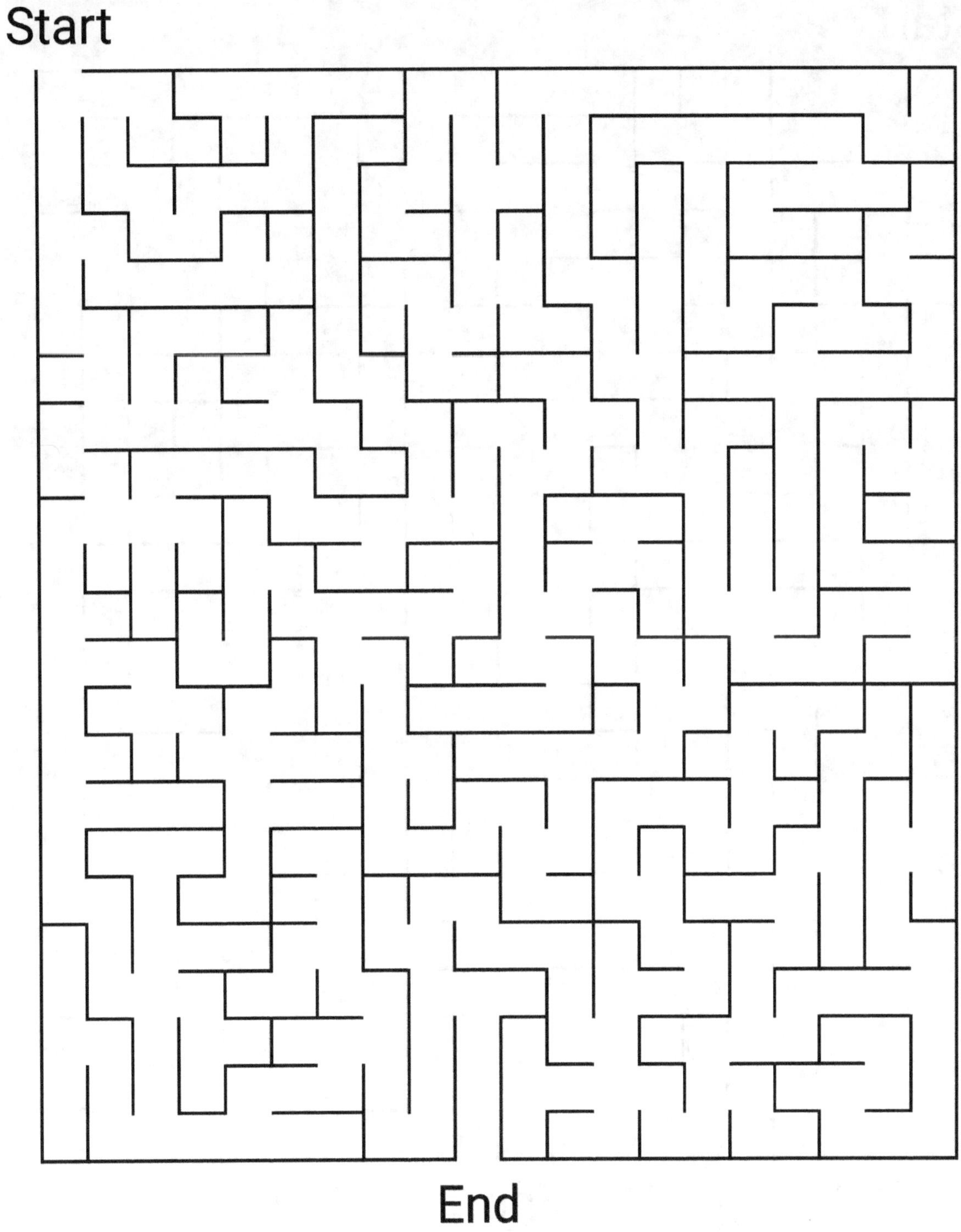

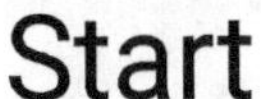

Start

End

Maze 5

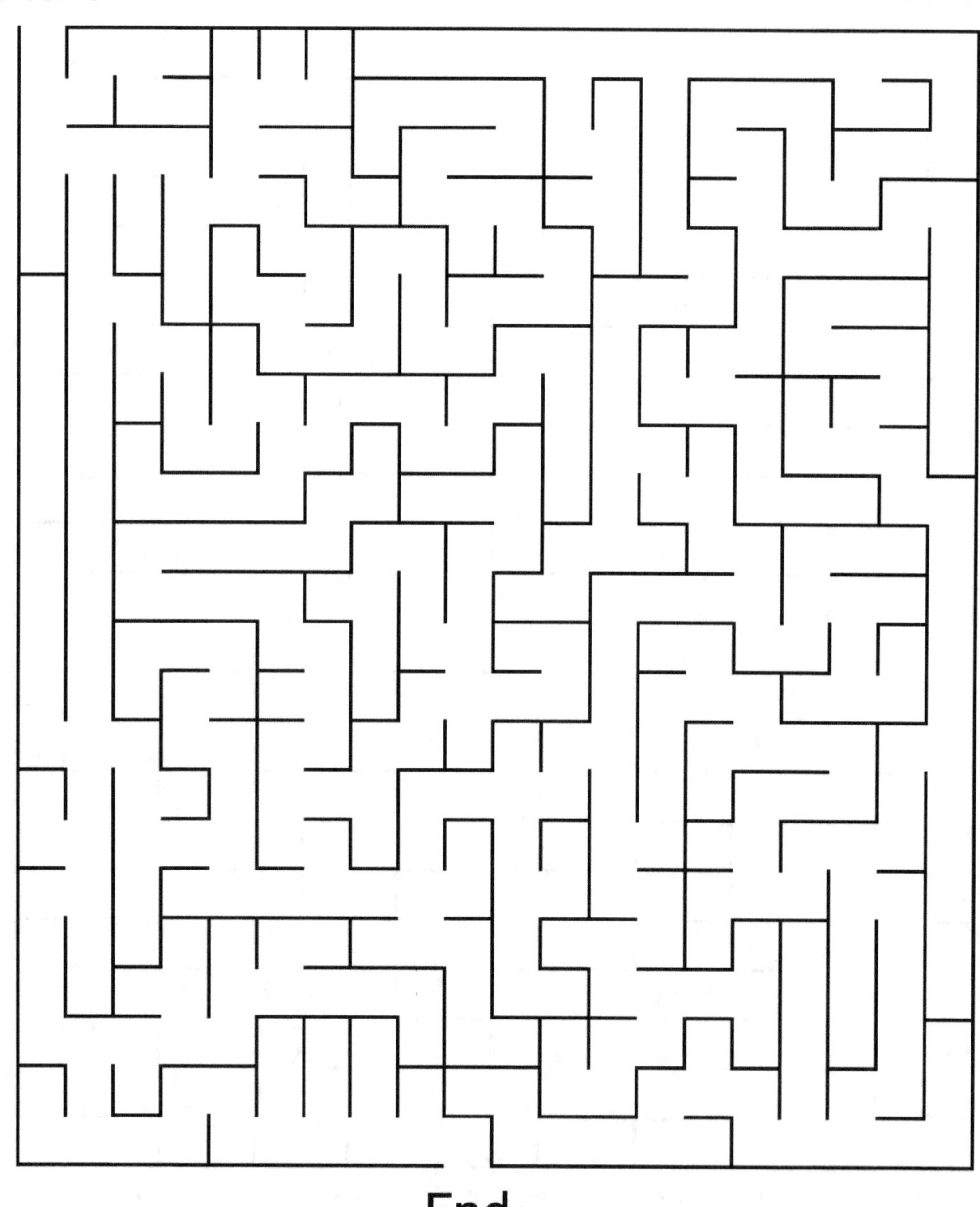

Maze 6

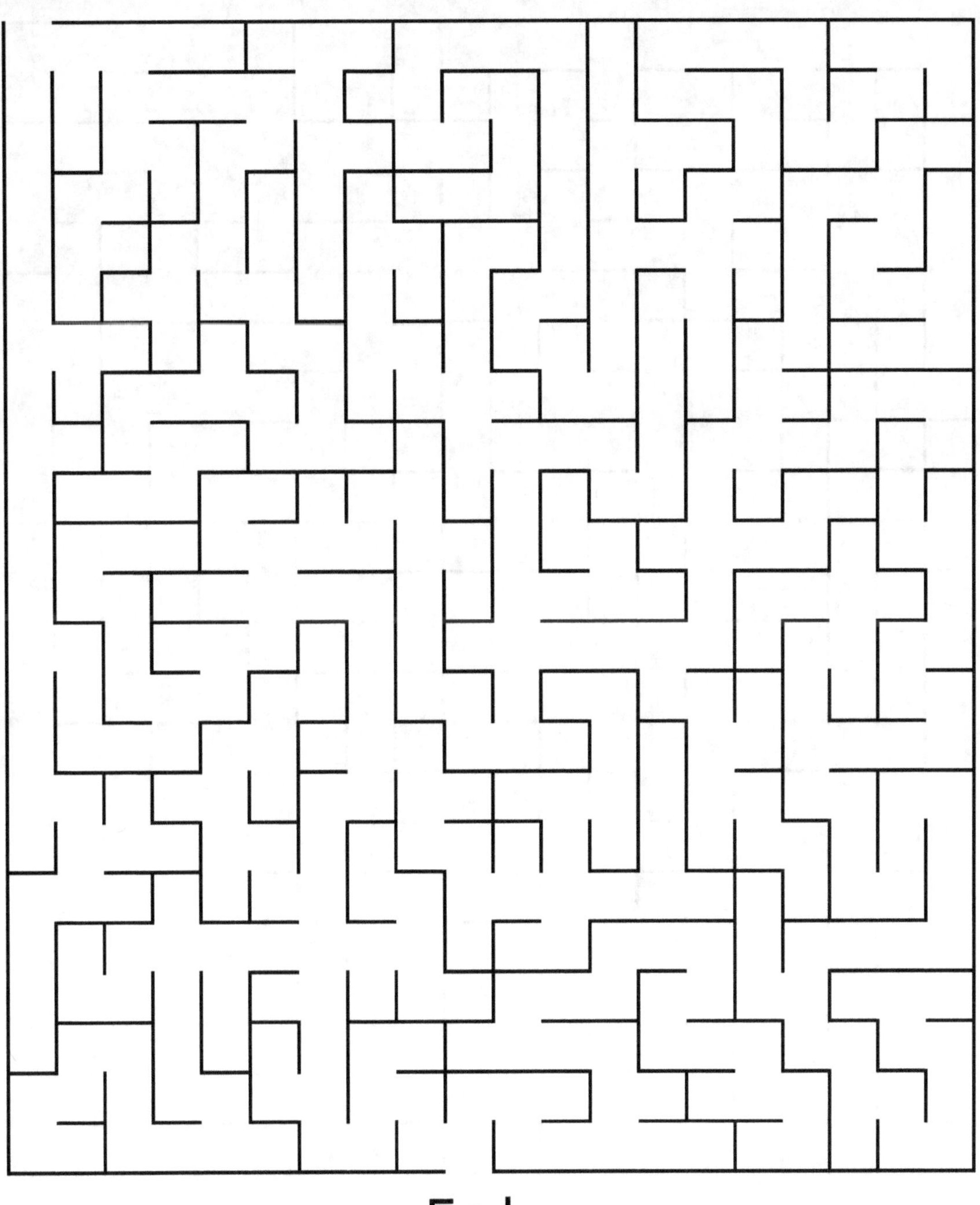

Maze 7

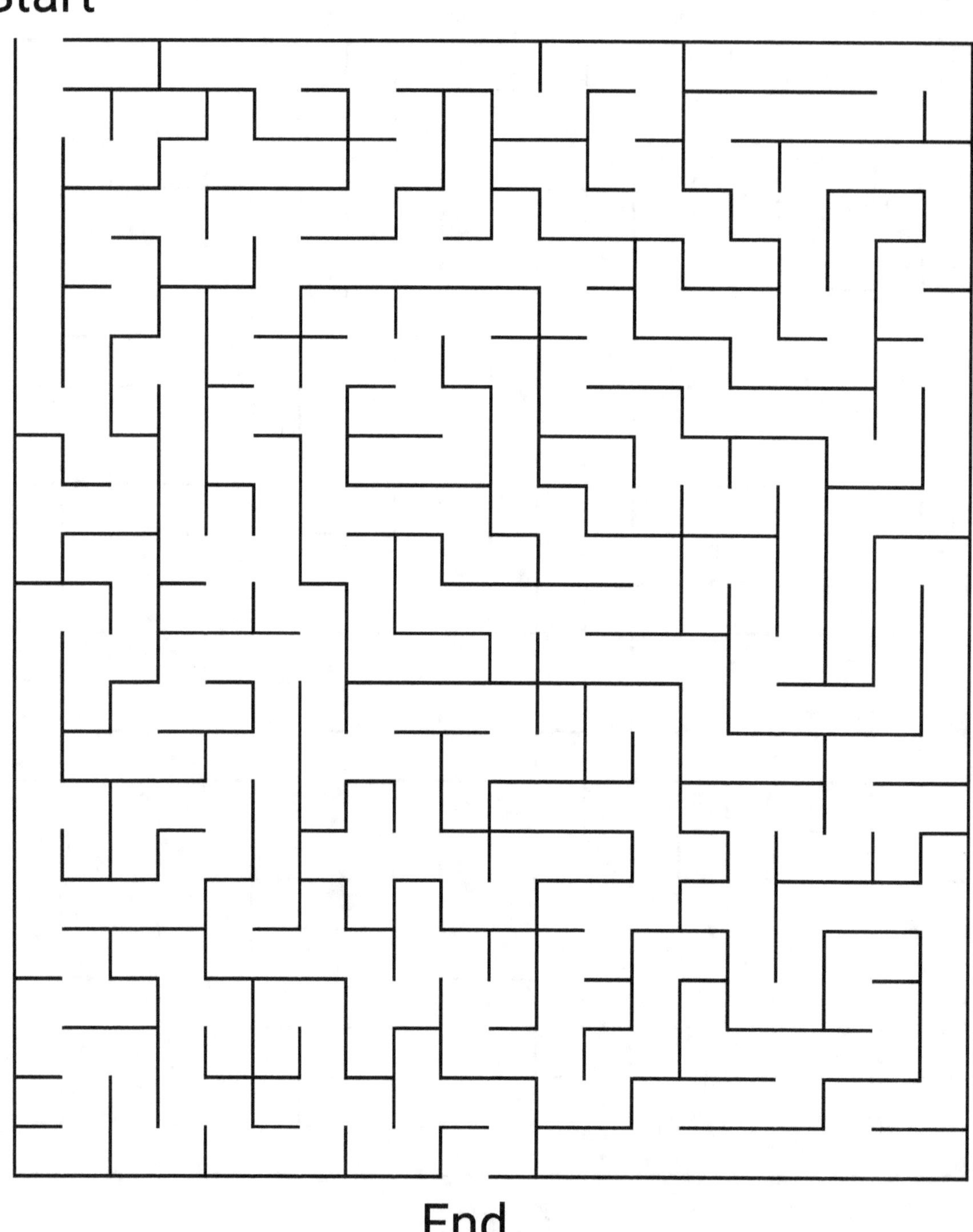

Maze 8

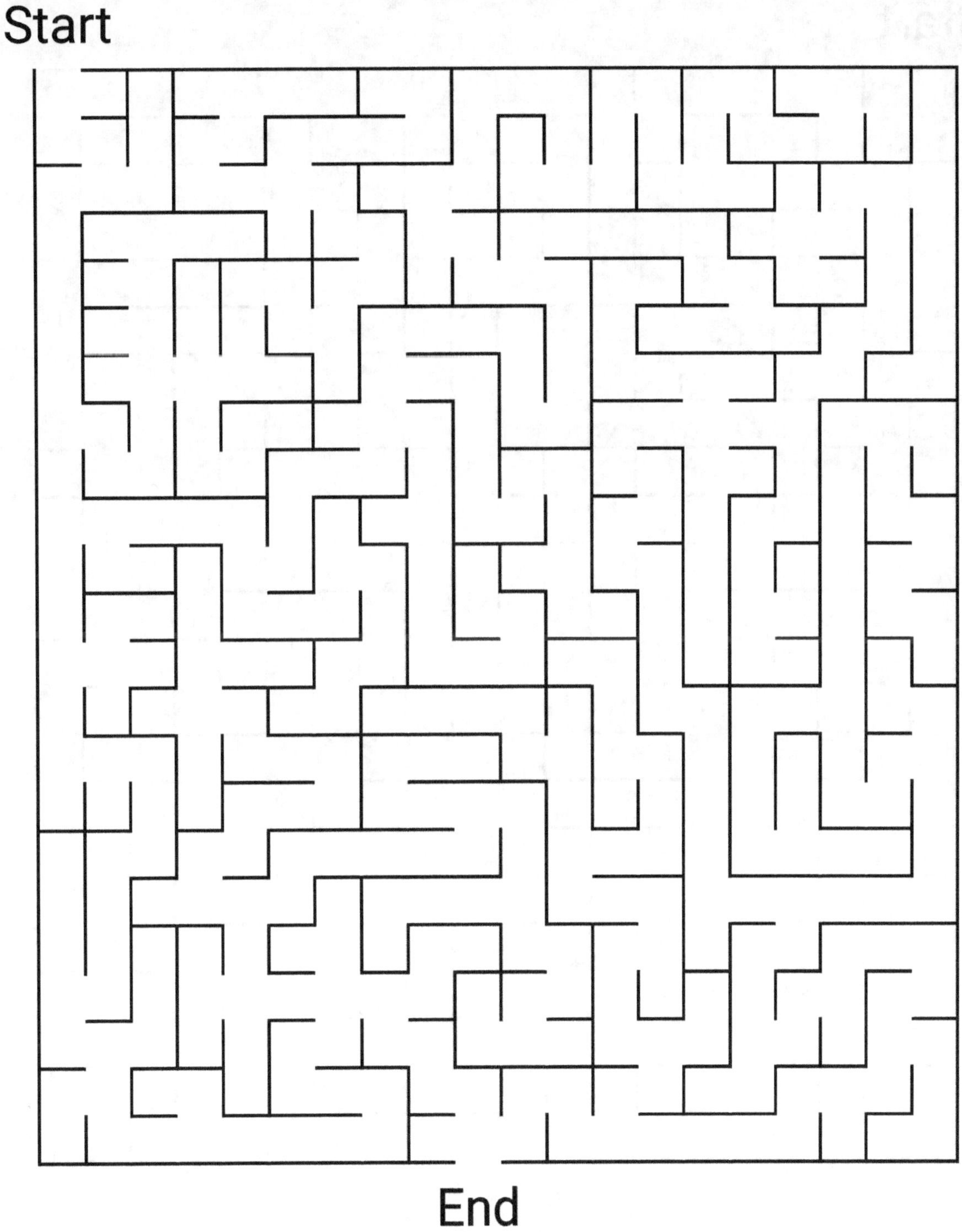

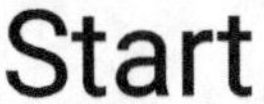

Maze 9

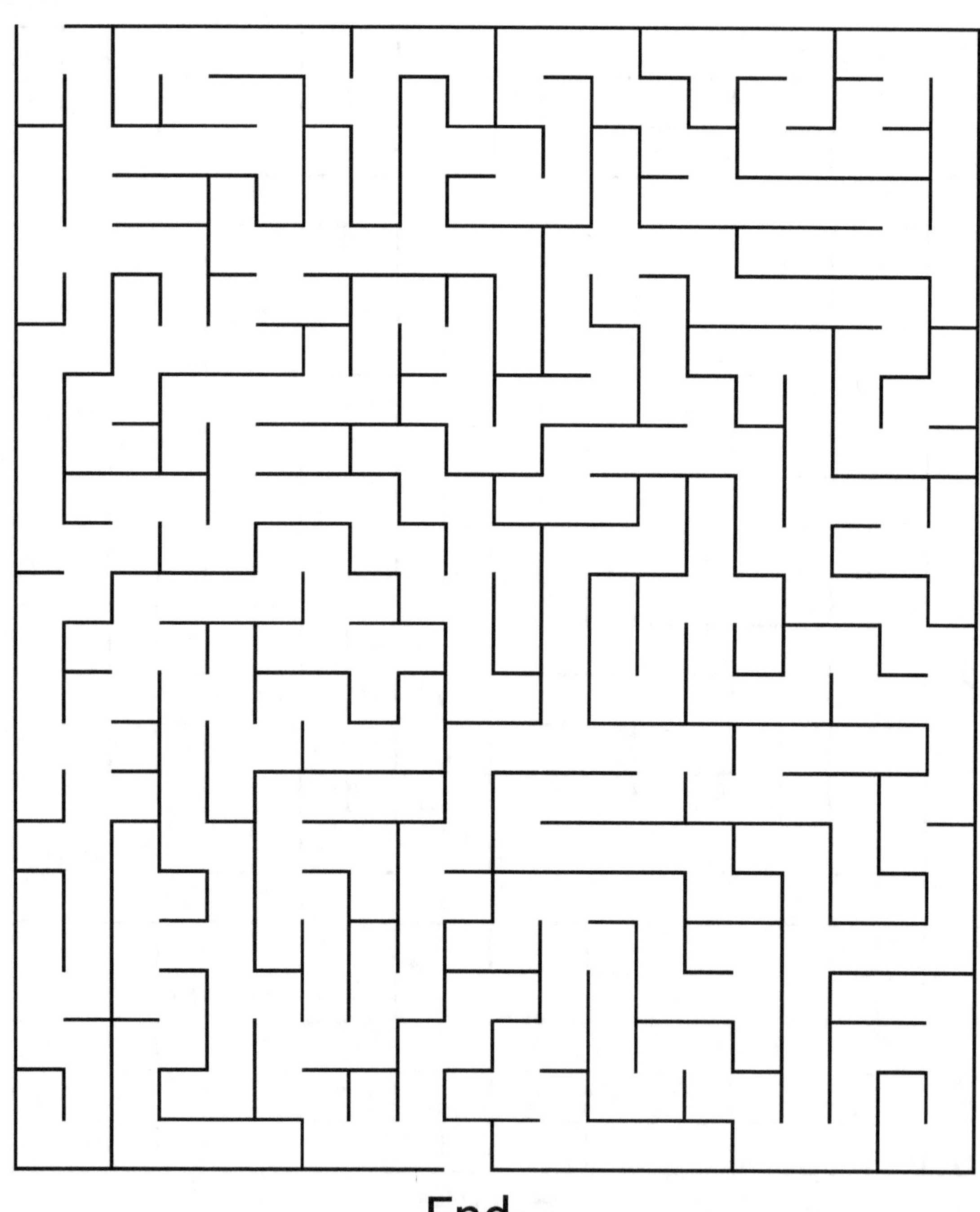

Maze 10

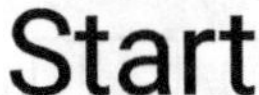

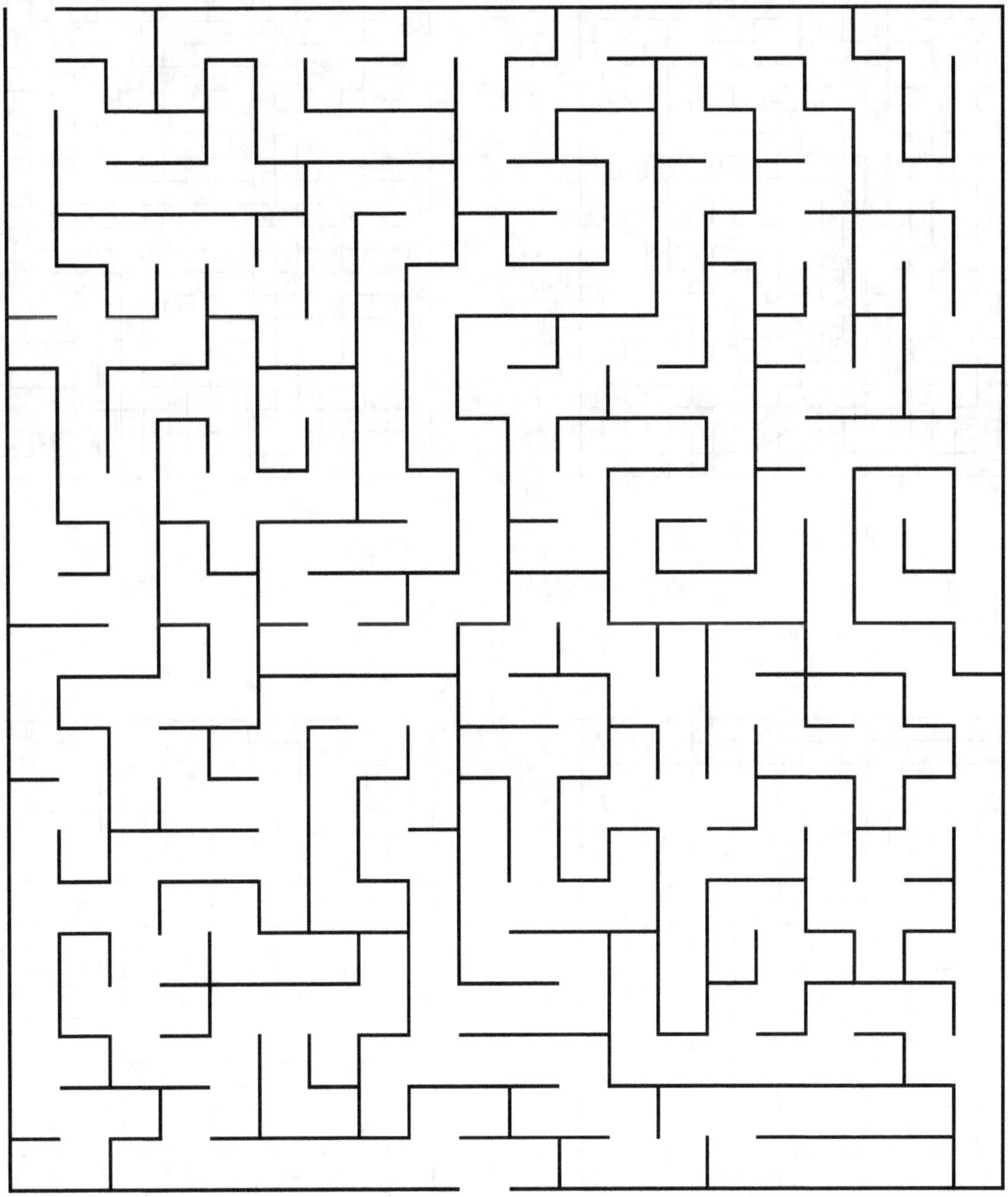

Mazes solutions

Maze 1

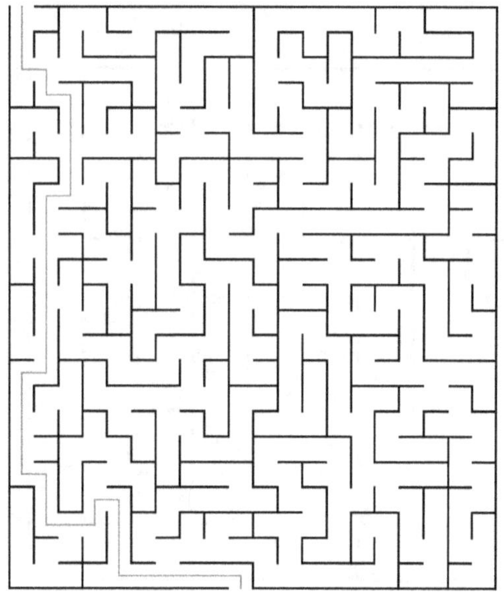

Maze 2

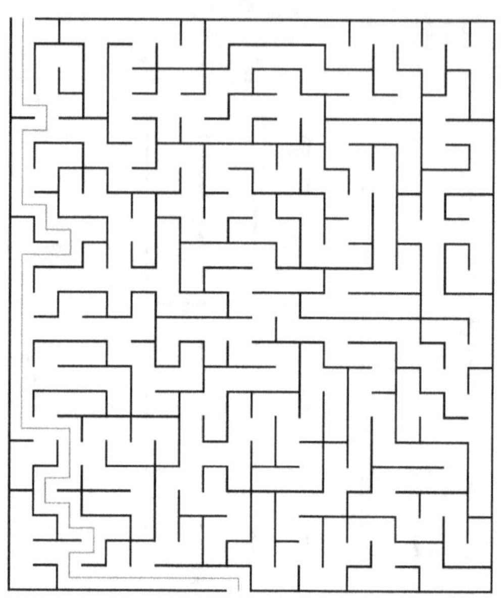

Maze 3

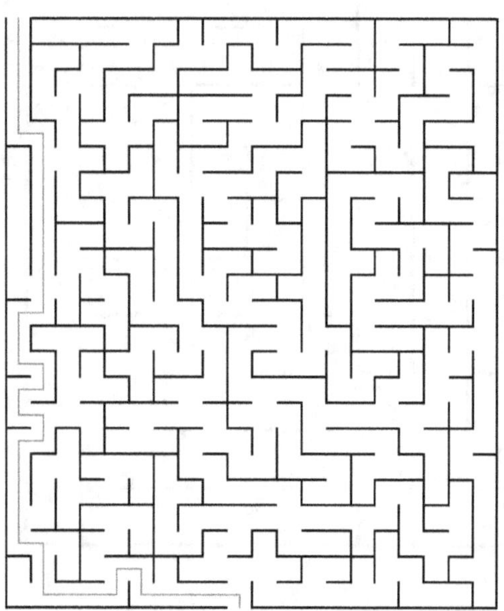

Maze 4

Mazes solutions

Maze 5

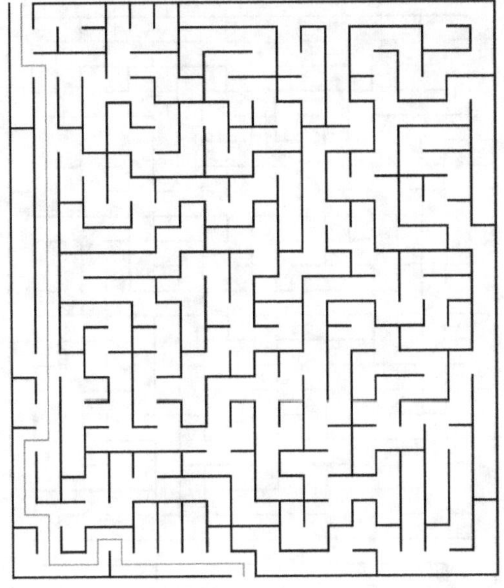

Maze 6

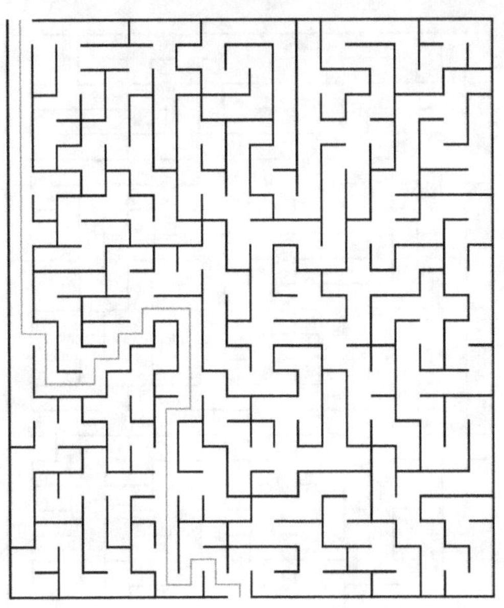

Maze 7

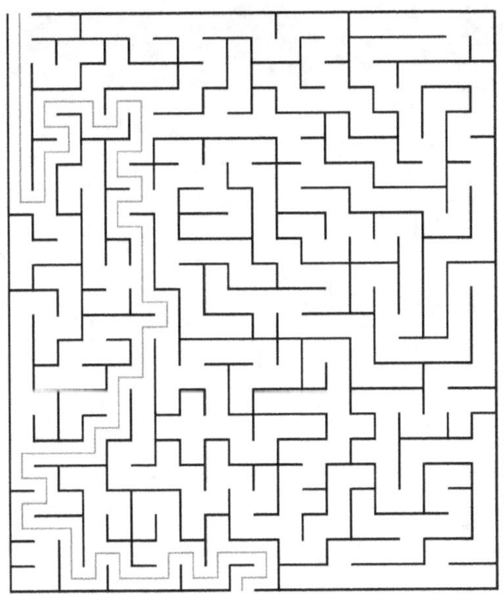

Maze 8

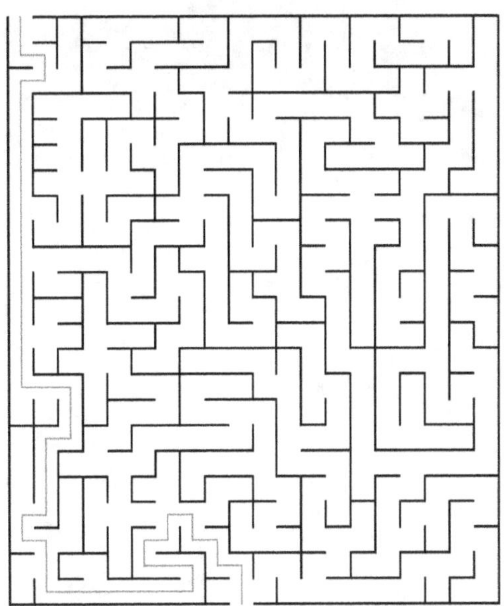

Mazes solutions

Maze 9

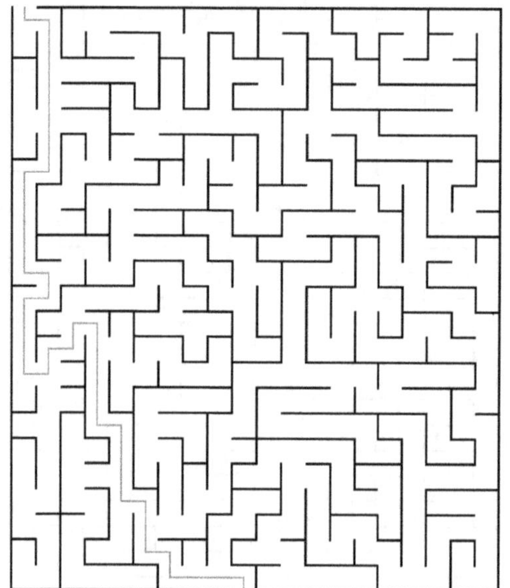

Maze 10

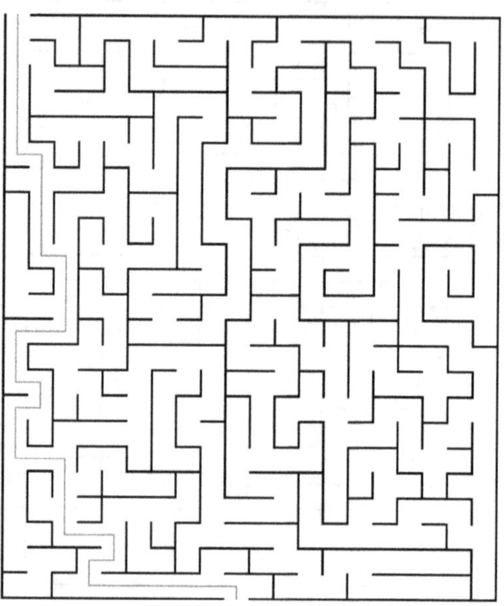

Word Scramble 1

IWHET = _______

DRE = _______

ERGEN = ______

EGRY = _______

EIOVLT = _______

WORNB = ______

NYVA = _______

LNMOE = ______

ABMRE = ______

CCHLOARA = ______

Word List

White	Red	Green
Grey	Violet	Brown
Navy	Lemon	Amber
Charcoal		

Word Scramble 2

ILVEO = _________

BRUY = _________

YIRVO = _________

MDRALEE = _________

BEUL = _________

RUTNBEET = _________

BCKLA = _________

OLEWYL = _________

YKS = _________

LUPREP = _________

Word List

Olive	Ruby	Ivory
Emerald	blue	Brunette
Black	Yellow	Sky
Purple		

Word Scramble 3

NAMGEAT = _________

PNKI = _________

UTESQOIRU = _________

RAGPE = _________

AES = _________

NZREOB = _________

YCNA = _________

ZERAU = _________

TGEANIENR = _________

SPIHPREA = _________

Word List

Magenta Pink Turquoise
Grape Sea Bronze
Cyan Azure Tangerine
Sapphire

Word Scramble 4

EREGN = _______

HAOCM = _______

RENAOG = _______

ELIM = ______

OSINMCR = _______

TADSRUM = _______

CRLAO = _______

TNA = _______

DEERALNV = ______

IGNDOI = _______

Word List

green	Mocha	Orange
Lime	Crimson	Mustard
Coral	Tan	Lavender
Indigo		

Word Scramble 5

ADRK = ______

ERAMC = ______

SLIVER = ______

IMTN = ______

ERRYHC = ______

DOROSOEW = ______

CEOEFF = ______

AHS = ______

OMNROA = ______

MLOSAN = ______

Word List

Dark	Cream	Silver
Mint	Cherry	Rosewood
Coffee	Ash	Maroon
Salmon		

Word Scramble 6

UQAA = ________

CPEHA = ________

RFNFOSA = ________

EALT = ________

BIEEG = ________

FAHUSIC = ________

NDRUUYBG = ________

VMUAE = ________

TRUS = ________

RLPAE = ________

Word List

Aqua	Peach	Saffron
Teal	Beige	Fuchsia
Burgundy	Mauve	Rust
Pearl		

Word Scramble 7

GENART = ________

LCLAI = ________

BURME = ________

LACETJBK = ________

CKHISRWA = ________

LAPERANI = ________

ECBCIYL = ________

KBIE = ________

RAENC = ________

ERRAGCAI = ________

Word List

Garnet	Lilac	Umber
Jet black	Rickshaw	Airplane
Bicycle	Bike	Crane
Carriage		

Word Scramble 8

ANV = _______

RRYFE = ______

ICLTOHREPE = _______

AECPJTK = _______

RROLY = ______

ERTOM = _______

WORAPYE = _______

YTOCSO = ______

TCAROTR = _______

TAE = _______

Word List

Van
Jetpack
Ropeway
Eat

Ferry
Lorry
Scooty

Helicopter
Metro
Tractor

Word Scramble 9

UACLNBAEM = ________

ABTO = ________

USB = ______

ACR = ______

EYLCC = ______

GROAC = ________

UCRTK = ______

ODNLAGOS = ______

OOUAHSBTE = ________

LESIMUNOI = ______

Word List

Ambulance	Boat	Bus
Car	Cycle	Cargo
Truck	Gondolas	Houseboat
Limousine		

Word Scramble 10

MCLYTEORCO = _________

ORWBTOA = _______

HIPS = _______

OOERTCS = _________

RTAIN = _______

RNIDK = _________

AEGEL = _______

CCEAKOP = _________

INOEGP = _______

ARKEEAPT = _________

Word List

Motorcycle   Rowboat   Ship
Scooter   Train   Drink
Eagle   Peacock   Pigeon
Parakeet

Word scramble solutions

Word Scramble 1

IWHET = WHITE

DRE = RED

ERGEN = GREEN

EGRY = GREY

EIOVLT = VIOLET

WORNB = BROWN

NYVA = NAVY

LNMOE = LEMON

ABMRE = AMBER

CCHLOARA = CHARCOAL

Word Scramble 2

ILVEO = OLIVE

BRUY = RUBY

YIRVO = IVORY

MDRALEE = EMERALD

BEUL = BLUE

RUTNBEET = BRUNETTE

BCKLA = BLACK

OLEWYL = YELLOW

YKS = SKY

LUPREP = PURPLE

Word Scramble 3

NAMGEAT = MAGENTA

PNKI = PINK

UTESQOIRU = TURQUOISE

RAGPE = GRAPE

AES = SEA

NZREOB = BRONZE

YCNA = CYAN

ZERAU = AZURE

TGEANIENR = TANGERINE

SPIHPREA = SAPPHIRE

Word Scramble 4

EREGN = GREEN

HAOCM = MOCHA

RENAOG = ORANGE

ELIM = LIME

OSINMCR = CRIMSON

TADSRUM = MUSTARD

CRLAO = CORAL

TNA = TAN

DEERALNV = LAVENDER

IGNDOI = INDIGO

Word scramble solutions

Word Scramble 5

ADRK = DARK

ERAMC = CREAM

SLIVER = SILVER

IMTN = MINT

ERRYHC = CHERRY

DOROSOEW = ROSEWOOD

CEOEFF = COFFEE

AHS = ASH

OMNROA = MAROON

MLOSAN = SALMON

Word Scramble 6

UQAA = AQUA

CPEHA = PEACH

RFNFOSA = SAFFRON

EALT = TEAL

BIEEG = BEIGE

FAHUSIC = FUCHSIA

NDRUUYBG = BURGUNDY

VMUAE = MAUVE

TRUS = RUST

RLPAE = PEARL

Word Scramble 7

GENART = GARNET

LCLAI = LILAC

BURME = UMBER

LACETJBK = JET BLACK

CKHISRWA = RICKSHAW

LAPERANI = AIRPLANE

ECBCIYL = BICYCLE

KBIE = BIKE

RAENC = CRANE

ERRAGCAI = CARRIAGE

Word Scramble 8

ANV = VAN

RRYFE = FERRY

ICLTOHREPE = HELICOPTER

AECPJTK = JETPACK

RROLY = LORRY

ERTOM = METRO

WORAPYE = ROPEWAY

YTOCSO = SCOOTY

TCAROTR = TRACTOR

TAE = EAT

Word scramble solutions

Word Scramble 9

UACLNBAEM = AMBULANCE

ABTO = BOAT

USB = BUS

ACR = CAR

EYLCC = CYCLE

GROAC = CARGO

UCRTK = TRUCK

ODNLAGOS = GONDOLAS

OOUAHSBTE = HOUSEBOAT

LESIMUNOI = LIMOUSINE

Word Scramble 10

MCLYTEORCO = MOTORCYCLE

ORWBTOA = ROWBOAT

HIPS = SHIP

OOERTCS = SCOOTER

RTAIN = TRAIN

RNIDK = DRINK

AEGEL = EAGLE

CCEAKOP = PEACOCK

INOEGP = PIGEON

ARKEEAPT = PARAKEET

Telling Time

Write the time inside each clock below

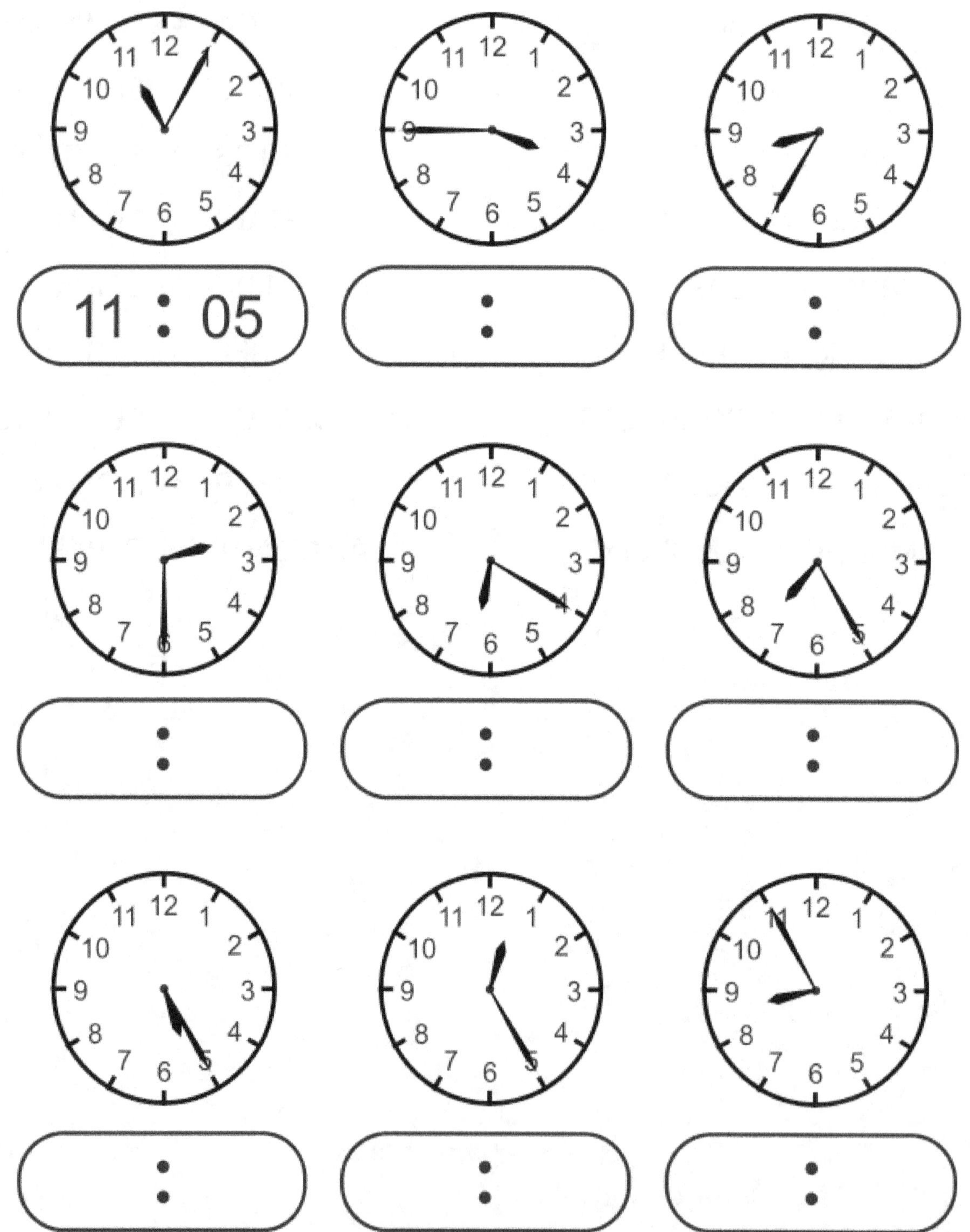

Telling Time

Write the time inside each clock below

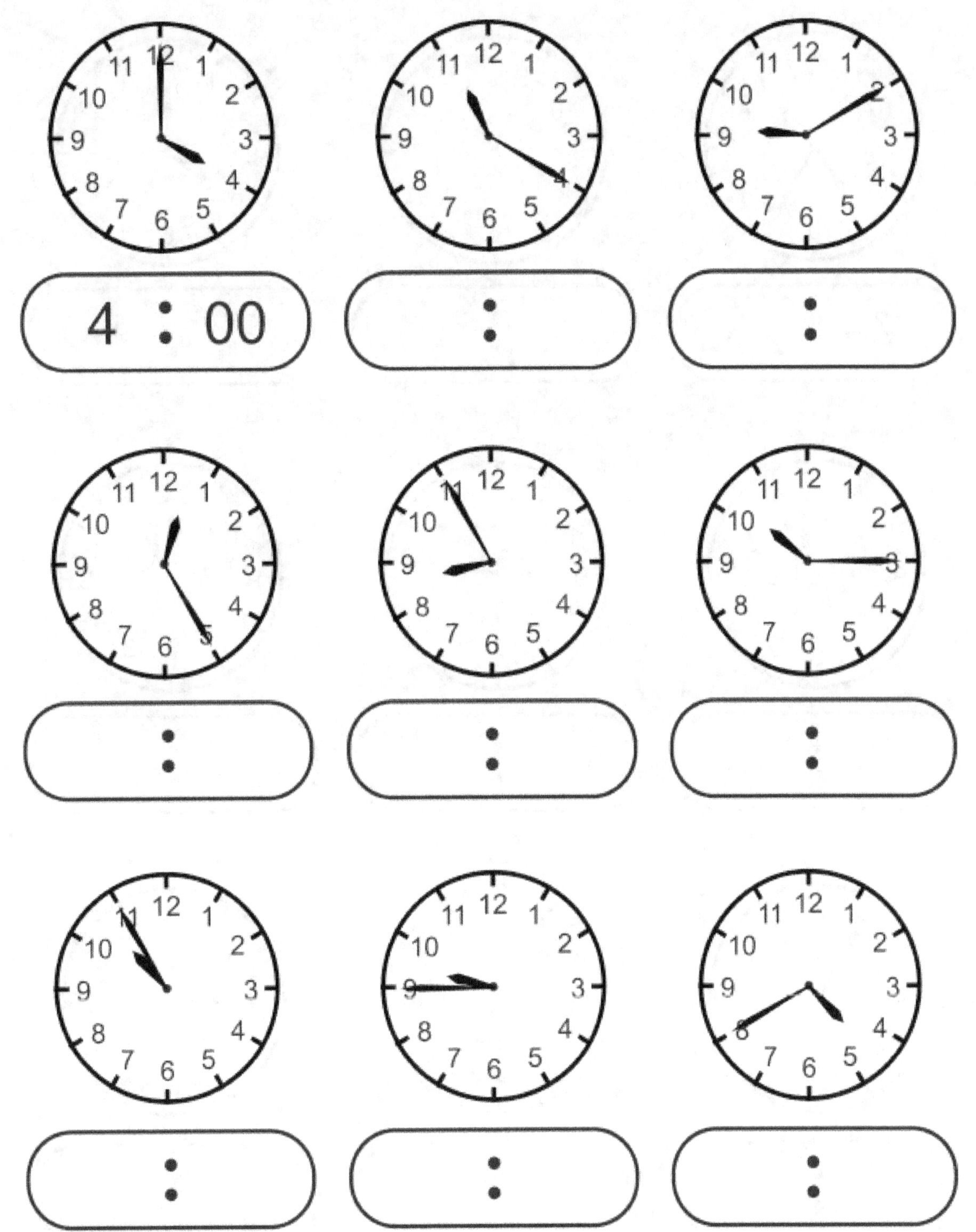

4 : 00

Telling Time

Write the time inside each clock below

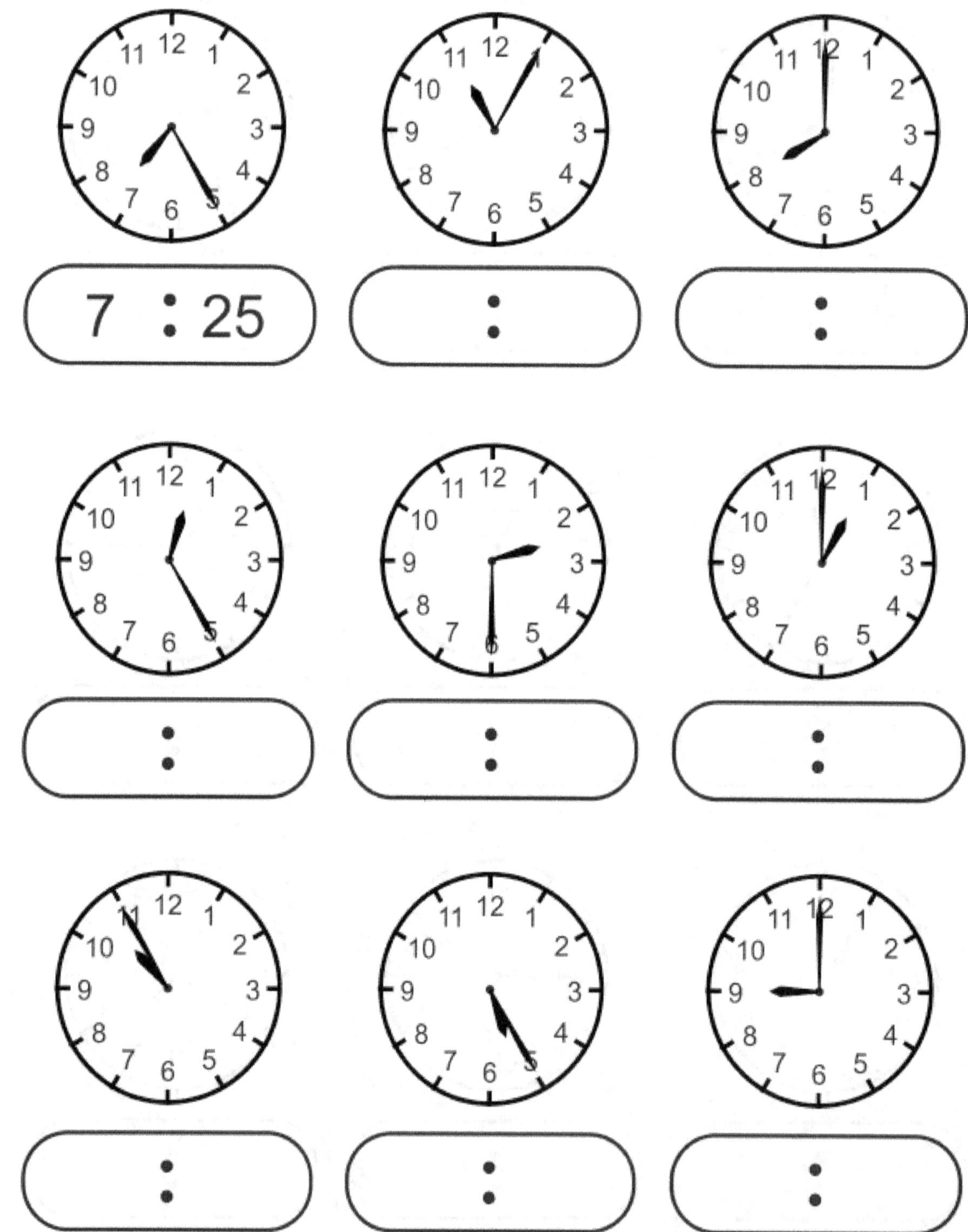

Telling Time

Write the time inside each clock below

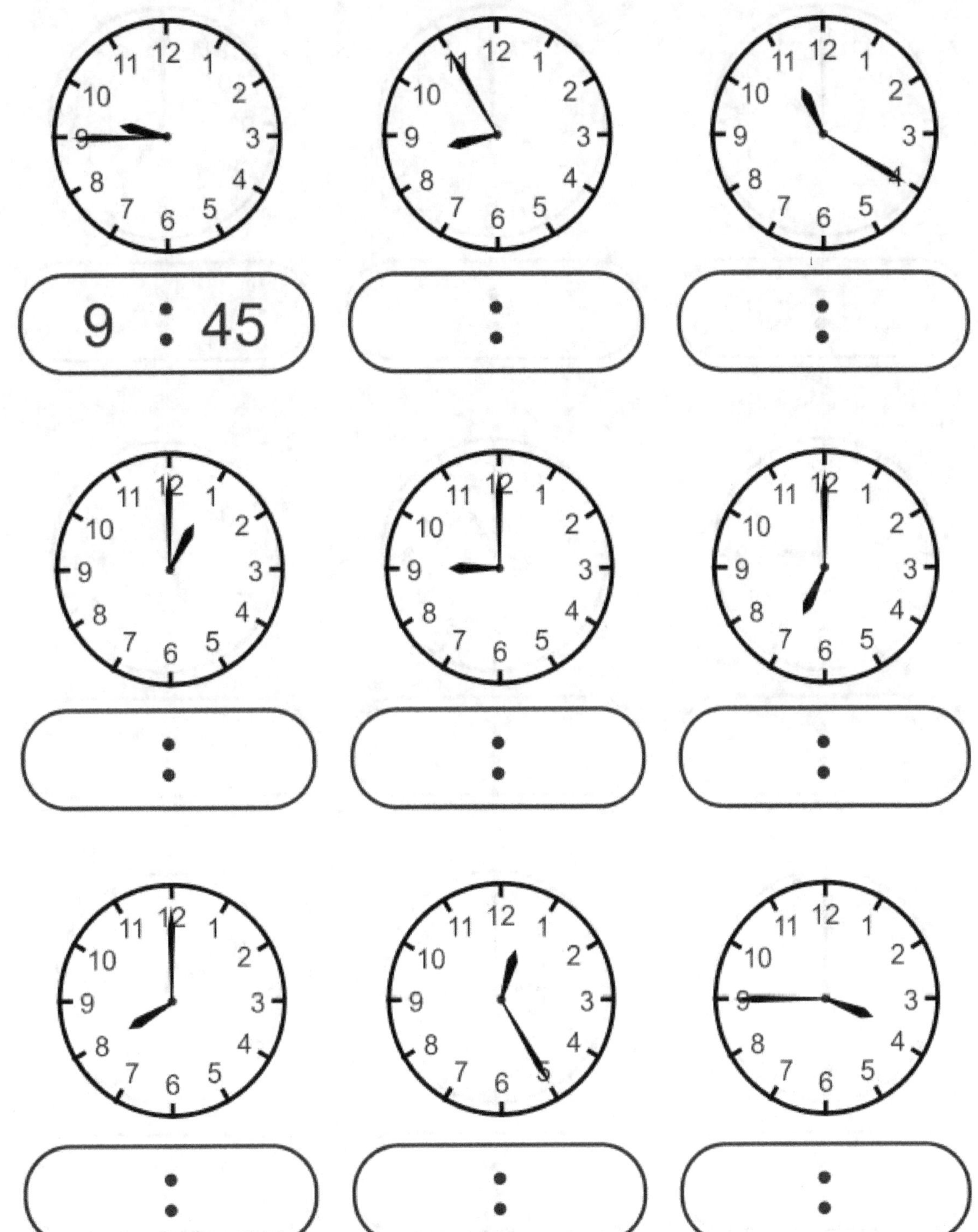

Telling Time

Write the time inside each clock below

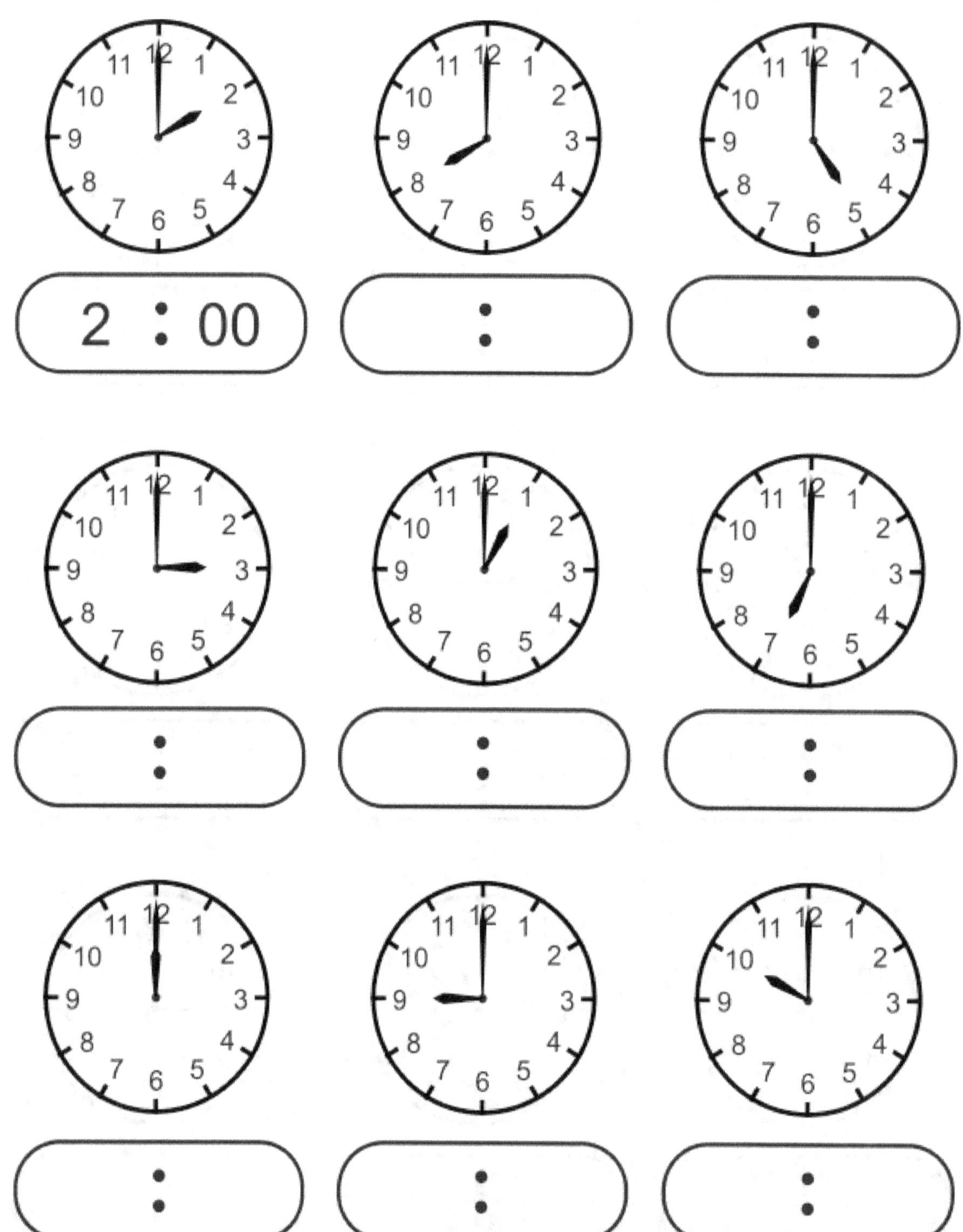

Telling Time

Draw a line to connect the matching times.

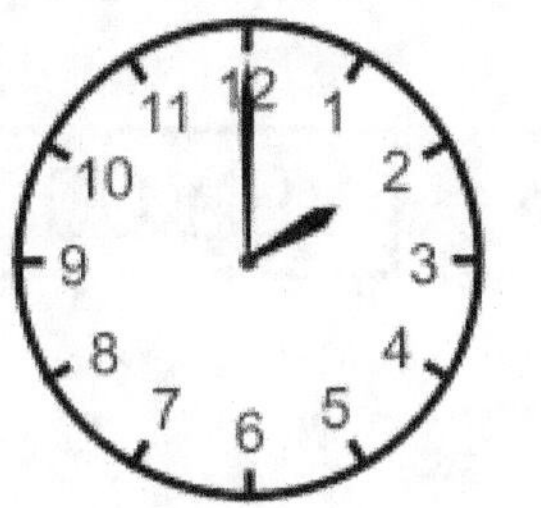 •   • 8 : 00

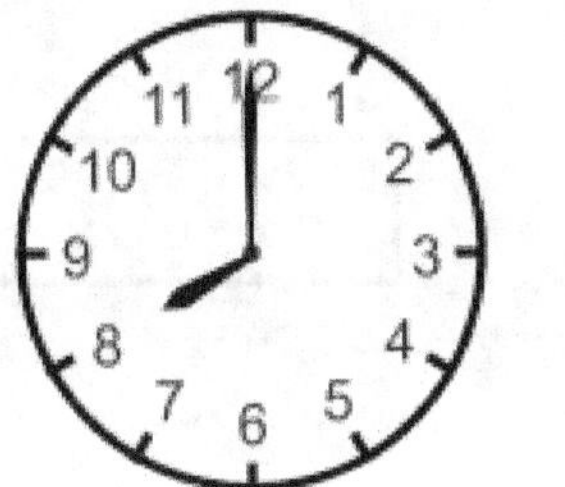 •   • 2 : 00

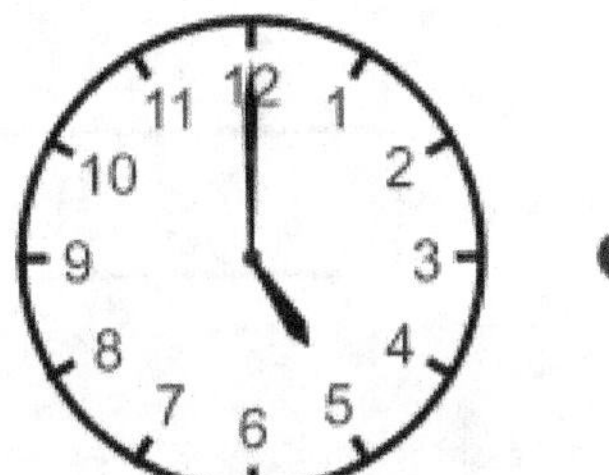 •   • 1 : 00

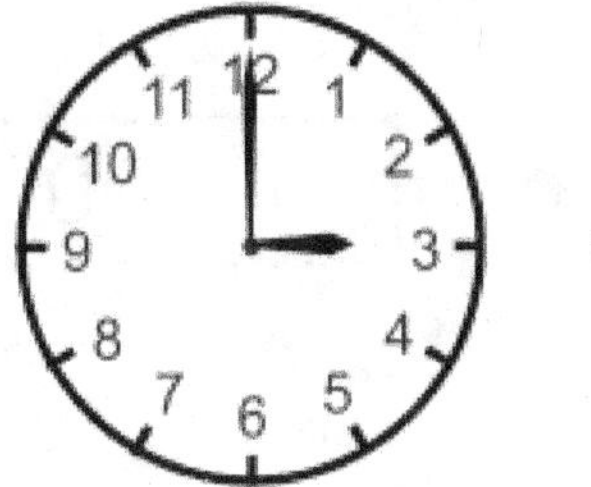 •   • 5 : 00

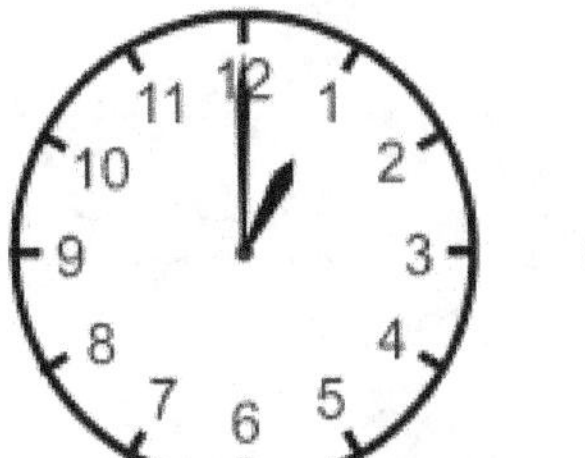 •   • 3 : 00

Telling Time

Draw a line to connect the matching times.

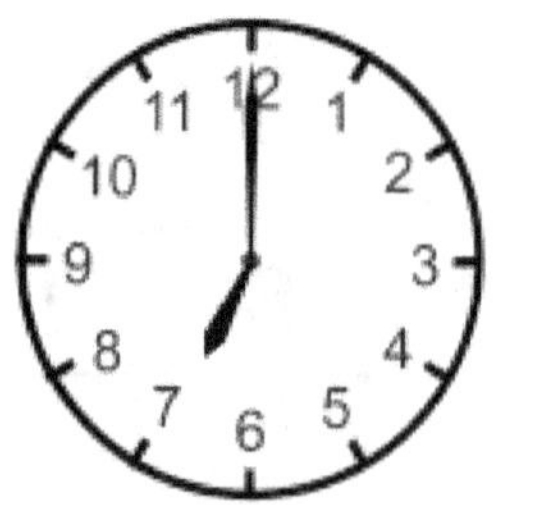

9 : 00

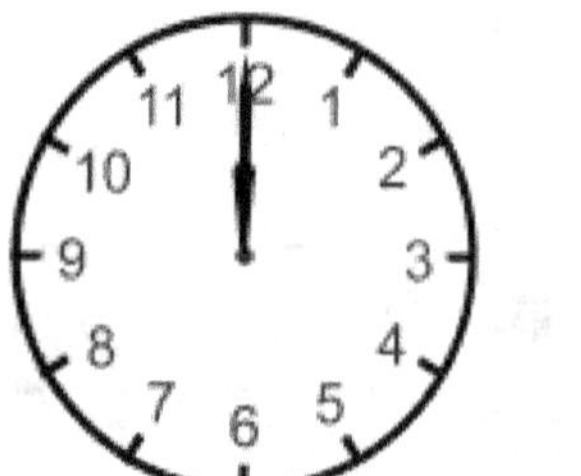

4 : 00

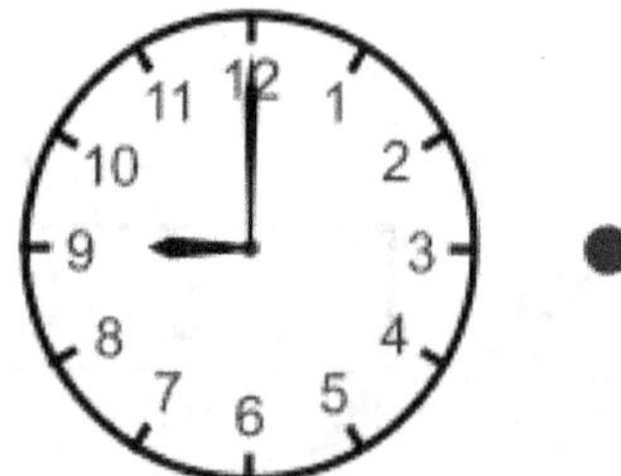

10 : 00

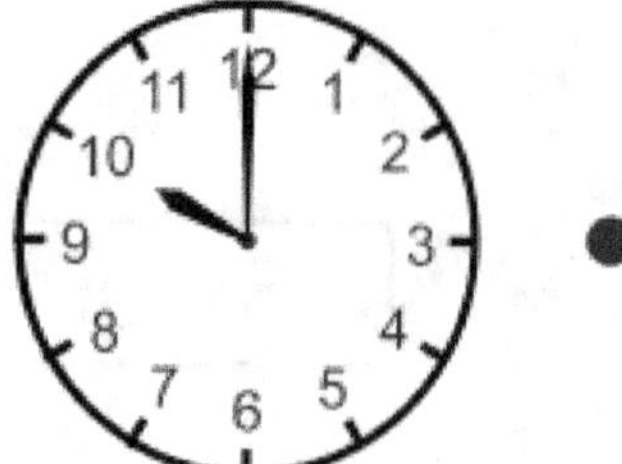

7 : 00

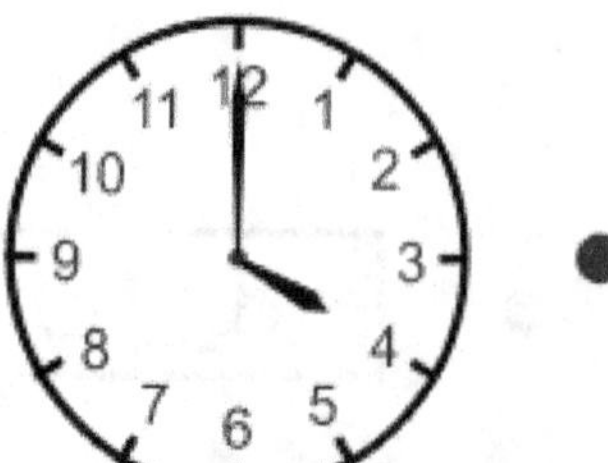

12 : 00

Sudoku 1

		6	3		
2	1	3			
6				3	
	4	5			
	6		5	4	3
5	3	4		2	6

Sudoku 2

6			1	5	
1	2			4	
3	6	2			5
	5	1	2	6	
5	4				
		6	5		

Sudoku 3

			5	1	2
	2				
2			4		3
	4	6		5	
6	1			4	5
5			1		6

Sudoku 4

	1				4
		4		3	1
6	4				5
		1			
4	6		1	2	3
1	2	3			6

Sudoku 5

				4	5
6				4	5
4			2	3	6
		3			2
5		6	3		
			5		1
2	5		4	6	

Sudoku 6

	3	4			5
6		1			4
4	1				3
			5	6	
5			4		1

Sudoku 7

	6	4			
3			4	6	
5					
				4	
1	5		3	2	
4	2			1	5

Sudoku 8

Sudoku 9

	1	3		5	
	4				3
				4	6
	5	6	2	3	
	2	5		1	
	6				

Sudoku 10

Sudoku 11

Sudoku 12

		3			6
	1	6		4	
6				3	
	4		2		5
			6		
		2	3	5	

Sudoku 13

		1	6	5	4
	5	4	1		
				4	
			5		
5	1				2
	6				5

Sudoku 14

Sudoku 15

Sudoku solutions

Sudoku 1

4	5	6	3	1	2
2	1	3	6	5	4
6	2	1	4	3	5
3	4	5	2	6	1
1	6	2	5	4	3
5	3	4	1	2	6

Sudoku 2

6	3	4	1	5	2
1	2	5	3	4	6
3	6	2	4	1	5
4	5	1	2	6	3
5	4	3	6	2	1
2	1	6	5	3	4

Sudoku 3

4	6	3	5	1	2
1	2	5	6	3	4
2	5	1	4	6	3
3	4	6	2	5	1
6	1	2	3	4	5
5	3	4	1	2	6

Sudoku 4

3	1	6	2	5	4
2	5	4	6	3	1
6	4	2	3	1	5
5	3	1	4	6	2
4	6	5	1	2	3
1	2	3	5	4	6

Sudoku solutions

Sudoku 5

6	3	2	1	4	5
4	1	5	2	3	6
1	4	3	6	5	2
5	2	6	3	1	4
3	6	4	5	2	1
2	5	1	4	6	3

Sudoku 6

2	3	4	6	1	5
6	5	1	3	2	4
3	2	5	1	4	6
4	1	6	2	5	3
1	4	3	5	6	2
5	6	2	4	3	1

Sudoku 7

2	6	4	1	5	3
3	1	5	4	6	2
5	4	1	2	3	6
6	3	2	5	4	1
1	5	6	3	2	4
4	2	3	6	1	5

Sudoku 8

2	6	5	4	1	3
3	1	4	6	2	5
5	2	1	3	6	4
4	3	6	2	5	1
1	4	2	5	3	6
6	5	3	1	4	2

Sudoku solutions

Sudoku 9

6	1	3	4	5	2
5	4	2	1	6	3
2	3	1	5	4	6
4	5	6	2	3	1
3	2	5	6	1	4
1	6	4	3	2	5

Sudoku 10

5	1	4	2	6	3
3	6	2	5	4	1
4	2	1	3	5	6
6	5	3	4	1	2
2	4	6	1	3	5
1	3	5	6	2	4

Sudoku 11

6	1	3	4	5	2
4	5	2	1	3	6
2	3	4	5	6	1
1	6	5	2	4	3
3	4	1	6	2	5
5	2	6	3	1	4

Sudoku 12

4	5	3	1	2	6
2	1	6	5	4	3
6	2	5	4	3	1
3	4	1	2	6	5
5	3	4	6	1	2
1	6	2	3	5	4

Sudoku solutions

Sudoku 13

3	2	1	6	5	4
6	5	4	1	2	3
1	3	5	2	4	6
2	4	6	5	3	1
5	1	3	4	6	2
4	6	2	3	1	5

Sudoku 14

6	5	4	1	3	2
1	3	2	4	6	5
5	1	6	2	4	3
2	4	3	5	1	6
4	6	5	3	2	1
3	2	1	6	5	4

Sudoku 15

6	4	5	1	2	3
2	1	3	5	6	4
1	2	4	3	5	6
3	5	6	4	1	2
5	3	2	6	4	1
4	6	1	2	3	5

Find two same pictures

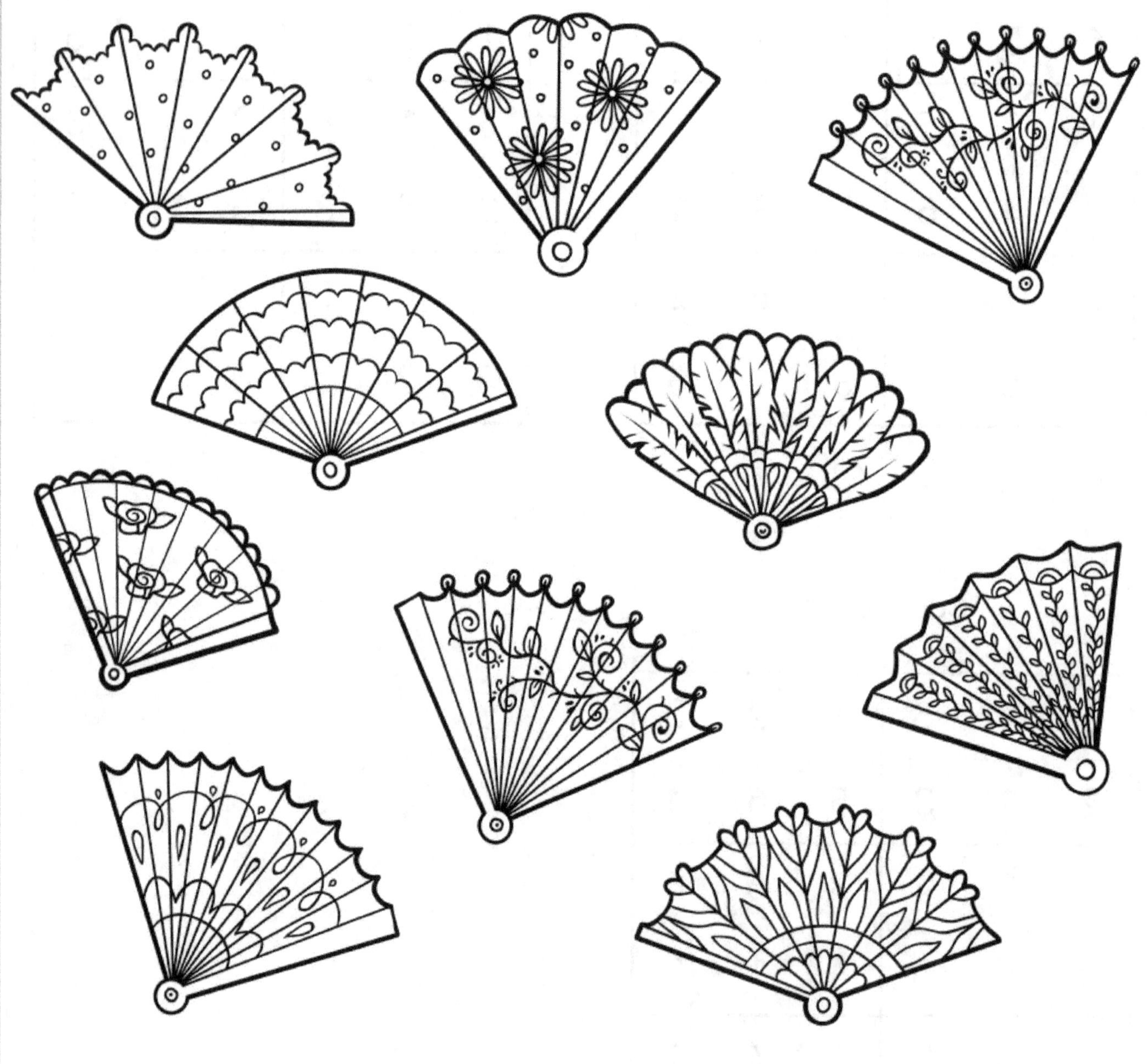

Find two same pictures

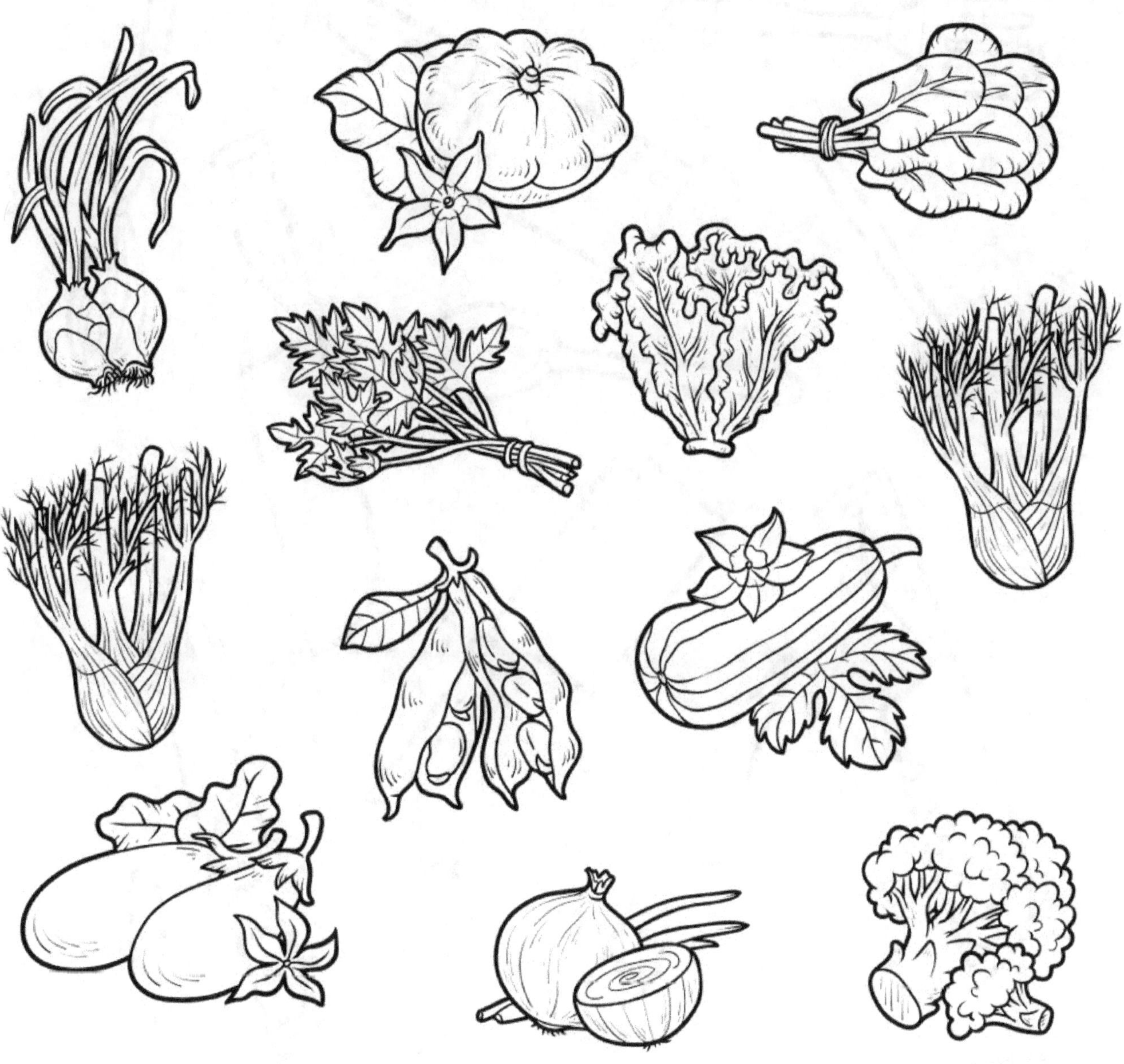

Find two same pictures

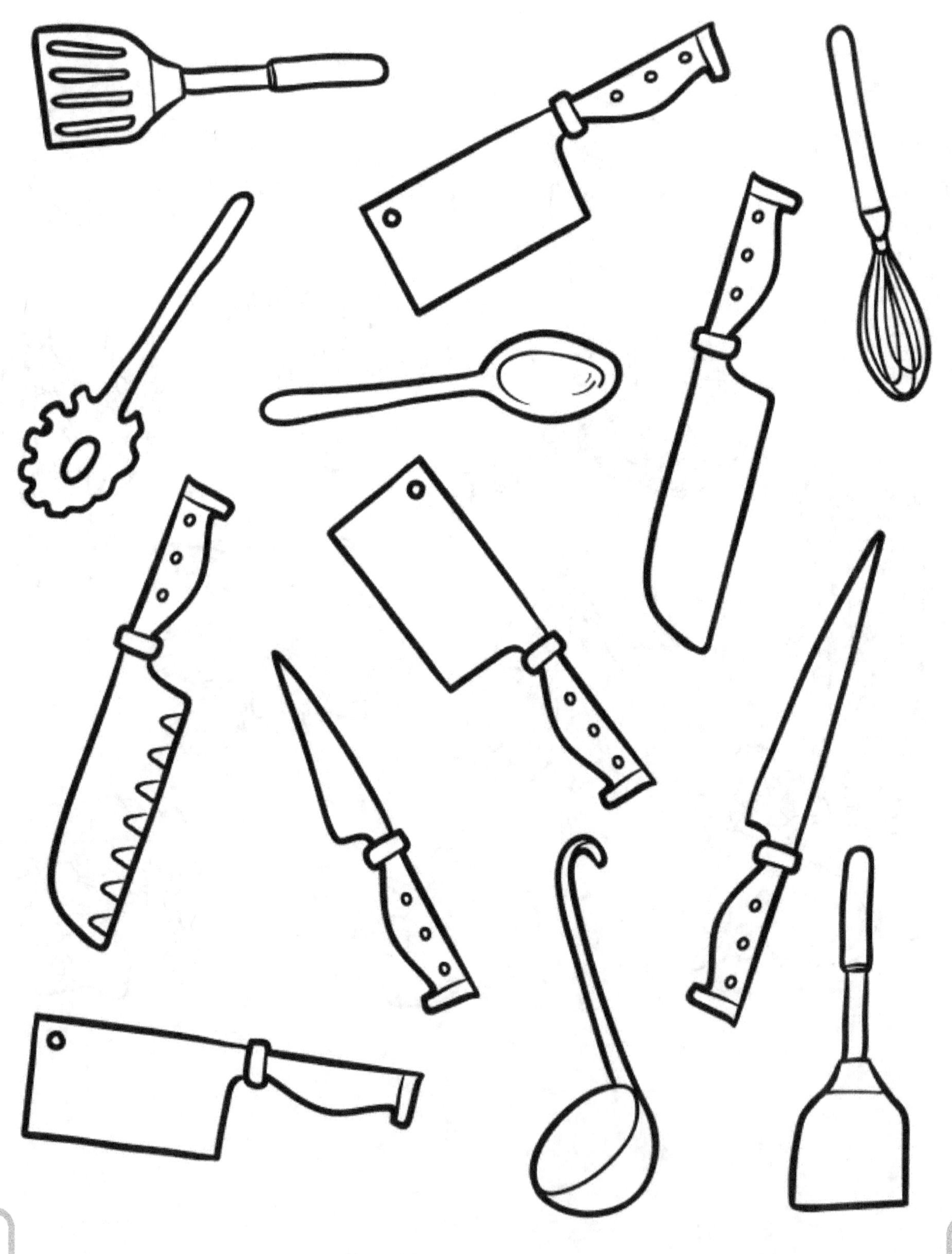

Find two same pictures

Find two same pictures

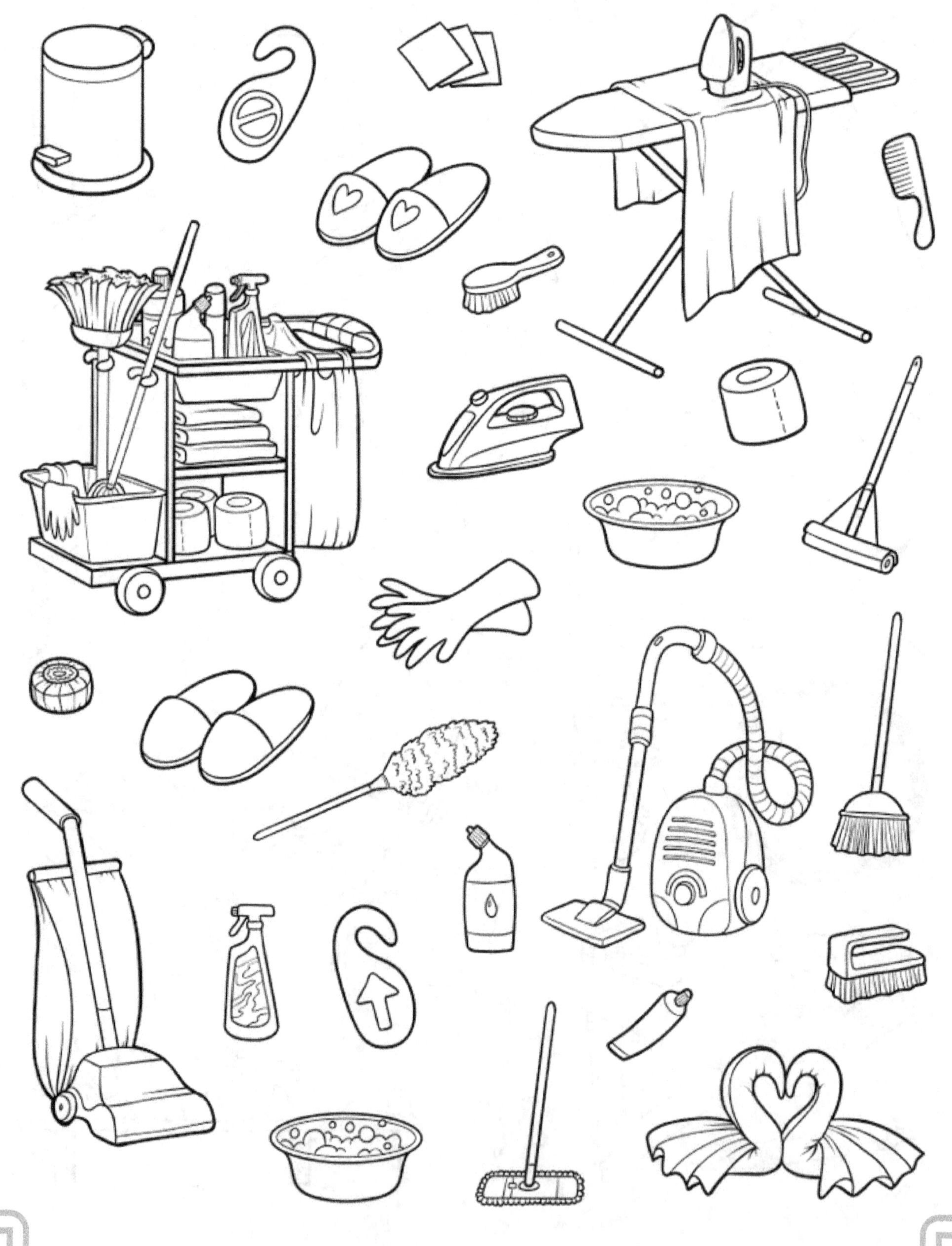

Find two same pictures

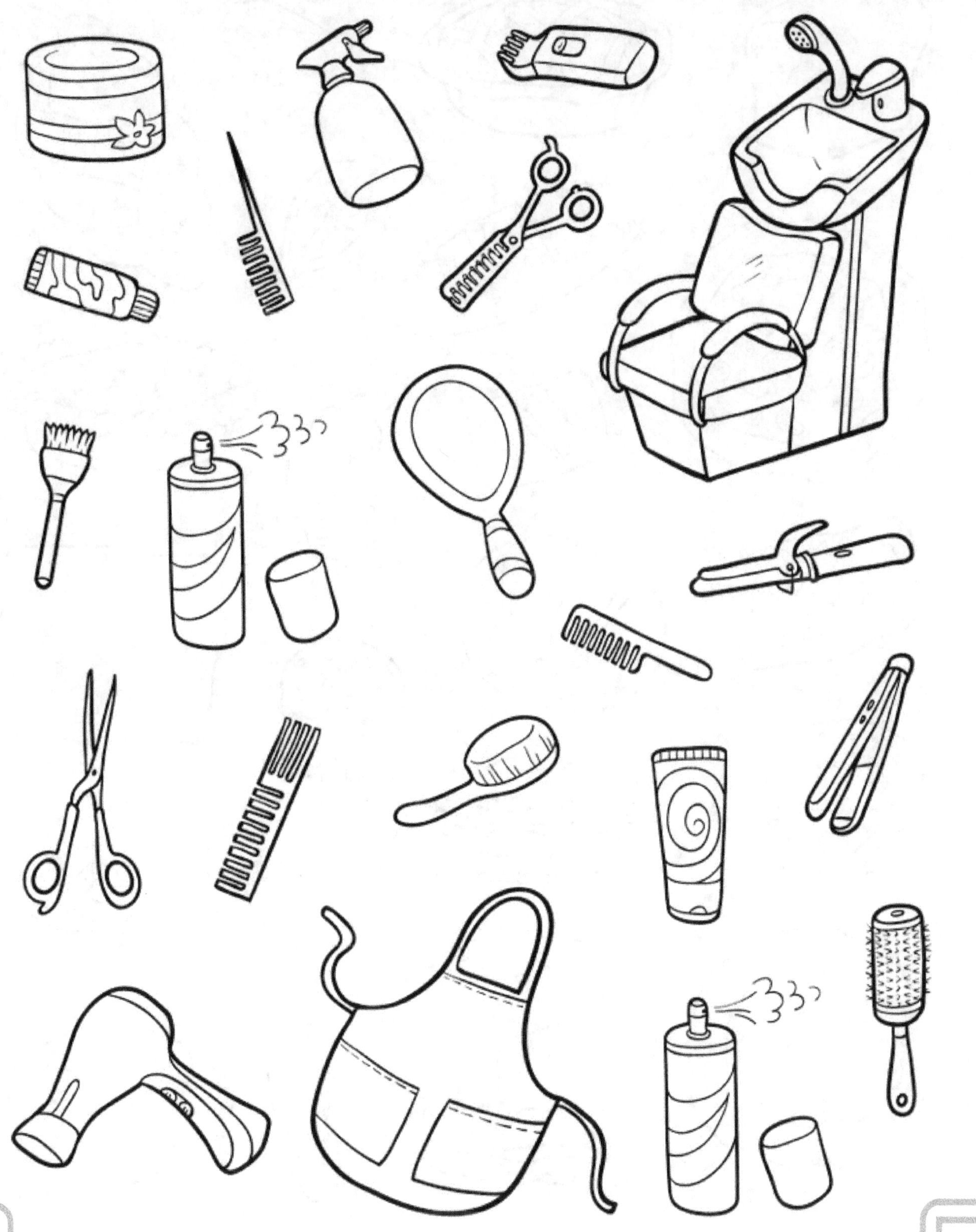

Find two same pictures

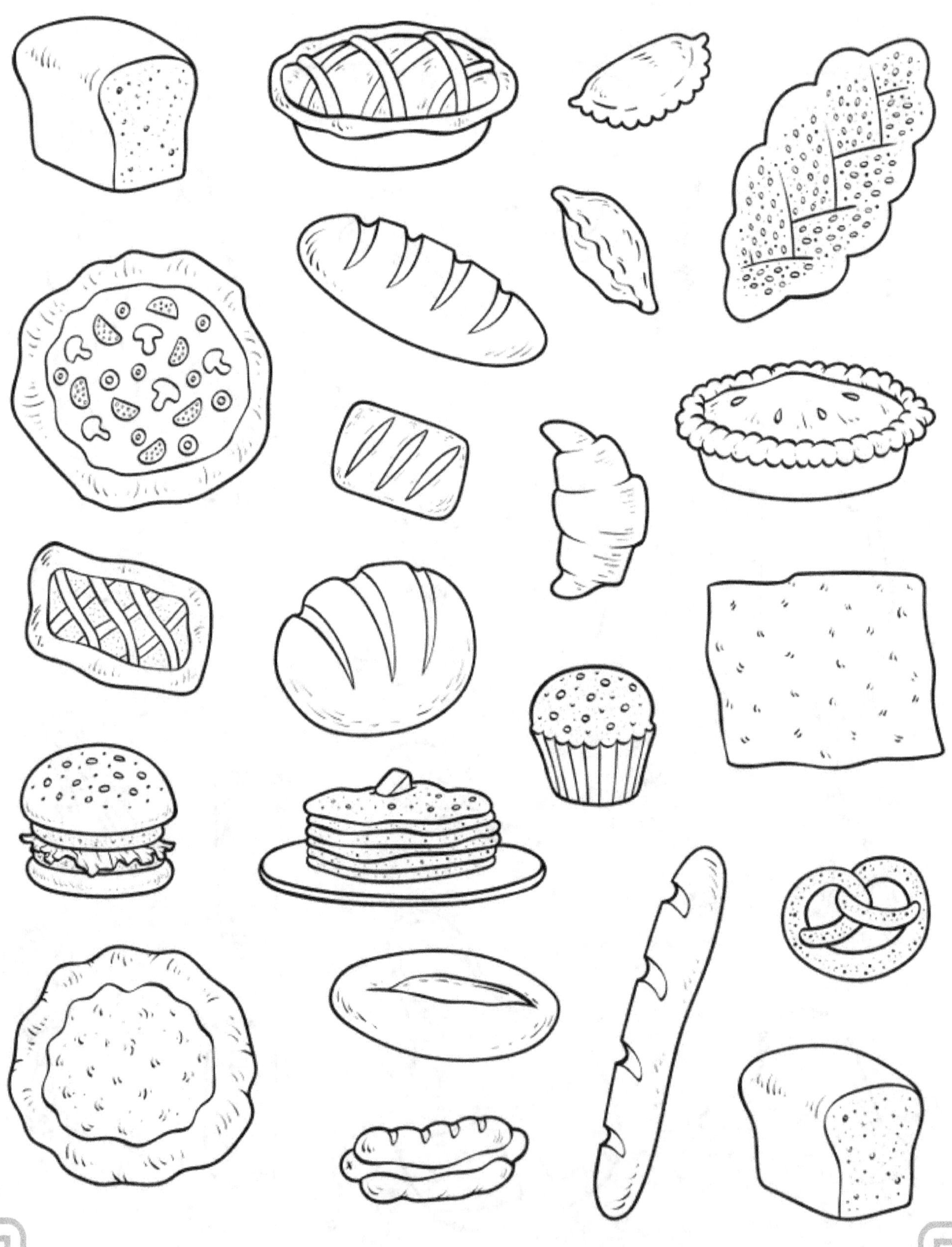

Find two same pictures

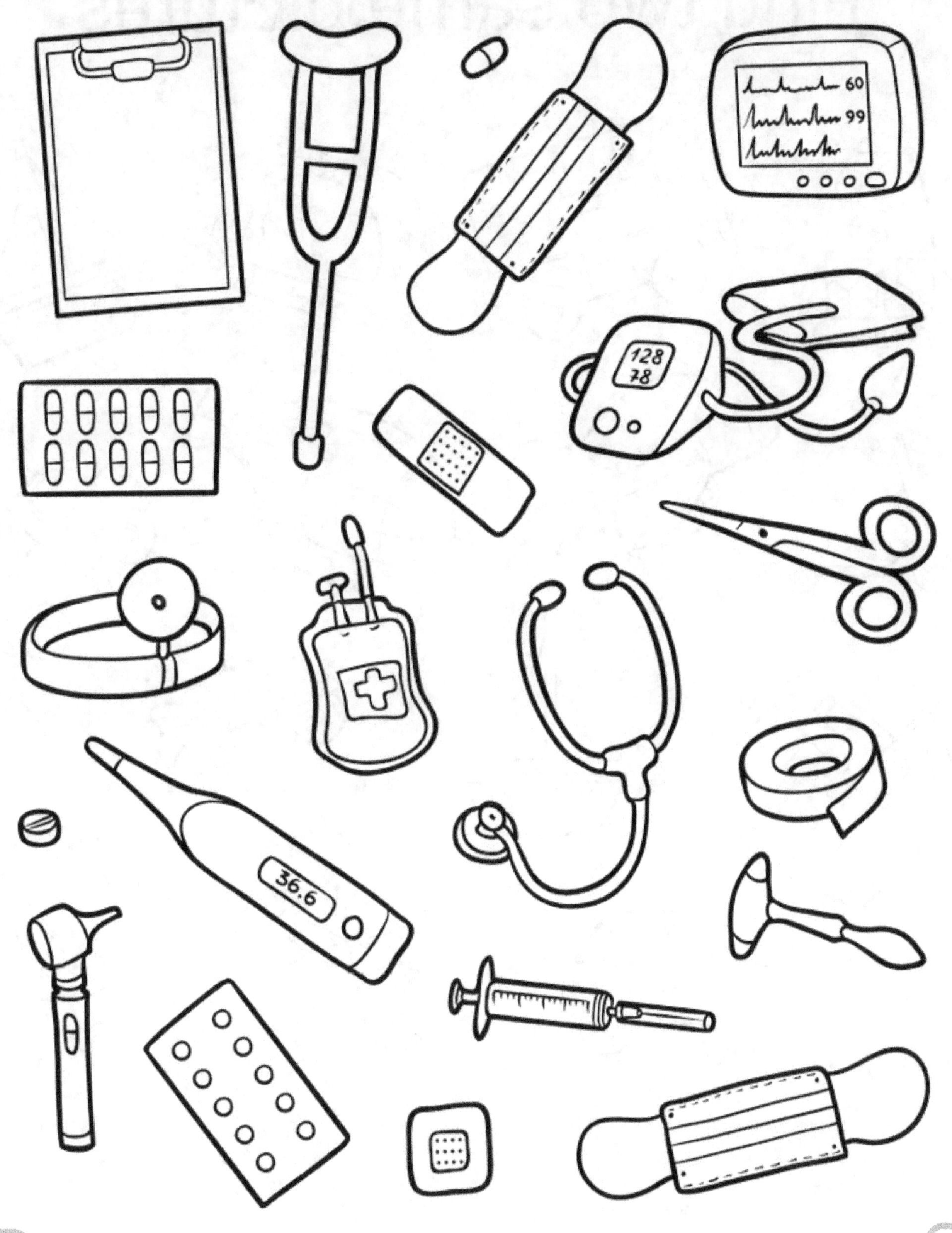

Find two same pictures

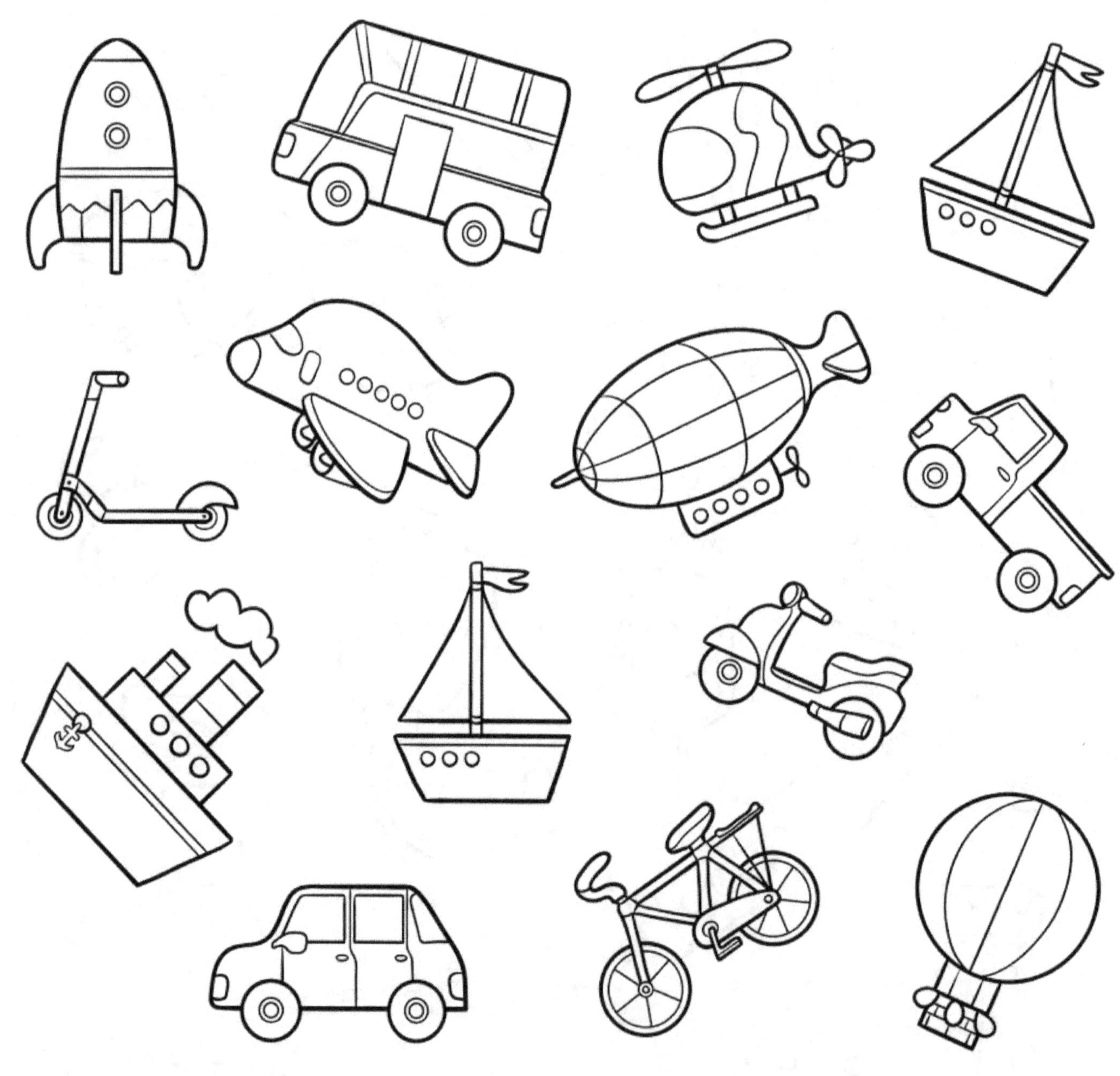

www.ingramcontent.com/pod-product-compliance
Lightning Source LLC
Chambersburg PA
CBHW081218260726
48653CB00010BB/3687